Crohn's Disease Cookbook

Essential Guide with 100 Recipes and a 30 Day Meal Plan for Better Health

Kate Princeton Johnson

Copyright 2020 by Kate Princeton Johnson- All rights reserved.

This document is geared towards providing exact and reliable information in regard to the topic and issue covered. The publication is sold on the idea that the publisher is not required to render an accounting, officially permitted, or otherwise, qualified services. If advice is necessary, legal or professional, a practiced individual in the profession should be ordered.

From a Declaration of Principles which was accepted and approved equally by a Committee of the American Bar Association and a Committee of Publishers and Associations.

In no way is it legal to reproduce, duplicate, or transmit any part of this document by either electronic means or in printed format. Recording of this publication is strictly prohibited and any storage of this document is not allowed unless with written permission from the publisher. All rights reserved.

The information provided herein is stated to be truthful and consistent, in that any liability, in terms of inattention or otherwise, by any usage or abuse of any policies, processes, or Directions: contained within is the solitary and utter responsibility of the recipient reader. Under no circumstances will any legal responsibility or blame be held against the publisher for any reparation, damages, or monetary loss due to the information herein, either directly or indirectly.

By continuing with this book, readers agree that the author is under no circumstances responsible for any losses, indirect or direct, that are incurred as a result of the information presented in this document, including, but not limited to inaccuracies, omissions and errors. Respective authors own all copyrights not held by the publisher. The information herein is offered for informational purposes solely and is universal as so. The presentation of the information is without a contract or any type of guarantee assurance.

The information herein is offered for informational purposes solely and is universal as so. The presentation of the information is without contract or any type of guarantee assurance. Readers acknowledge that the author is not engaging in the rendering of legal, financial, medical or professional advice. Please consult a licensed professional before attempting any techniques outlined in this book.

Contents

Are Crohn's Disease, Inflammatory Bowel Disease and 8
Ulcerative Colitis all the same? 8
    Inflammatory Bowel Disease 8
Crohn's Disease Explained 14
Crohn's Disease and the Stress Connection 23
    A Body Weighed Down By Stress 23
    How do our bodies cope with stress? 23
    A Deeper Look at Inflammation 25
Starting the Healing Process 30
    Inflammation and Stress Explained 30
    Effective Ways of Healing Crohn's Disease Symptoms 32
Crohn's Disease Eating Recap 43
Part Two: CHRON'S-TREATMENT MEAL PLAN & RECIPES 45
30-DAY CHRON'S DIET MEAL PLAN 45
CHRON'S DIET BREAKFAST RECIPES 52

1. Gut-Healing Chocolate Breakfast Shake 52
2. Chia Seed & Peanut Butter Protein Pudding 53
3. Healthy Avocado & Berry Acai Smoothie 54
4. Spring Onion & Salmon Frittata 55
5. Chai-Cashew Latte Oatmeal 57
6. Gut-Healing Ginger Pineapple Juice 59
7. Detox Oatmeal Porridge 60
8. Shrimp & Avocado Omelet 61
9. Coconut Yogurt Peanut Butter Parfait 63
10. Healthy Whole Food Breakfast Smoothie 64
11. Cheesy Red Onion Omelet 65

12.	Healthy Berry Breakfast Shake	67
13.	Ginger and Red Onion Pancakes	68
14.	Gut-Healing Smoothie	70
15.	Salmon Omelet	71
16.	Turmeric Almond Milk & Berry Shake	72
17.	Superfood Breakfast Bowl	73
18.	Healing Green Smoothie	74
19.	Scrambled Eggs & Grilled Salmon with Avocado	75
20.	Herbs Omelet	77
21.	Ginger Berry Anti-Inflammatory Smoothie	78
22.	Peanut Butter Chocolate Swirl Porridge	79
23.	Mushroom & Tomato Omelet	81
24.	Healthy Coconut Pancakes	83
25.	Healthy Breakfast Casserole	85
26.	Ginger Detox Smoothie	87
27.	Spicy Breakfast Carrot Pudding	88

CHRON'S DIET LUNCH RECIPES		90
28.	Spinach & Turkey Soup	90
29.	Healthy Beef Lettuce Wraps	92
30.	Healthy Savory Beef Stew	94
31.	Shrimp & Pineapple Curry	95
32.	Lean Steak & Veggie in Coconut Curry Sauce	97
33.	Healthy Protein-Packed Fish Tikka Curry	99
34.	Protein Chicken Curry with Coconut Rice	101
35.	Gut Healing Soup	103
36.	Delicious Low Carb Chicken Curry	105
37.	Zucchini & Mushroom Soup	107
38.	Lettuce Avocado & Egg Salad Wraps	109

39.	Grilled Shiitake Mushrooms	111
40.	Healthy Savory Beef Stew with Avocado	112
41.	Italian Fish Stew with Yummy Mashed Potatoes	114
42.	Lean Steak & Mung Cleansing Soup	116
43.	Sauteed Green Bean & Zucchini Bowl	118
44.	Lemony Squash Salad	120
45.	Tasty Bean Soup with Tortilla Chips	122
46.	Vegan Red Lentil Soup	124
47.	Lunch Salad with Lemony Dressing	126
48.	Chickpea Salad Wrap	128
49.	Mango & Grilled Steak Salad w/ Buttermilk-Avocado Buttermilk Dressing	130
	Tasty Lime Cilantro Cauliflower Rice	132
50.	Turmeric Chickpea & Artichoke Sauté	134
51.	Crunchy Salmon Arugula Salad	136
52.	Delicious African Beef Curry	138
	CHRON'S DIET DINNER RECIPES	140
53.	Sweet Potato & Herbed Chicken Casserole	140
54.	Chili Fried Steak with Toasted Cashews	142
55.	Grilled Chicken with Fresh Herb Marinade	144
56.	Salmon Served with Mashed Potatoes	146
57.	Grilled Steak Salad with Red Onion, Orange & Avocado	148
58.	Super Tasty Mushroom Marinara with Pasta	150
59.	Stir Fried Beef with Veggies	152
60.	Creamy Citrus Salmon Baked in Coconut Milk	154
61.	Tilapia with Mushroom Sauce	156
62.	Spiced Roast Side of Salmon	158
63.	Curried Prawns with White Bread	160

64.	Hot Lemon Garlic Prawns with Rice	162
65.	White Fish & Coconut Rice	164
66.	Grilled Beef & White Rice	166
67.	Ginger Chicken with Veggies	168
68.	Tasty Coconut Cod	170
69.	Lemon BBQ Salmon	172

CHRON'S DIET SNACKS/DESSERTS..................................174

70.	Juice for Gut Health	174
71.	Raw Banana Mash Snack	175
72.	Stomach Soothing Juice	176
73.	Sautéed Kale with Citrus Sauce	177
74.	Orange & Aloe Vera Juice	178
75.	Chocolaty Kamut Energy Bars	179
76.	Gut Friendly Smoothie	181
77.	Delicious Mashed Lime Peas	182
78.	Green Peanut Butter Smoothie	184
79.	Delicious Humus	185
80.	Easy and Tasty Pumpkin Muffin in a Cup	187
81.	Detoxifying Turmeric Tea	188
82.	Green Fruit Drink	190
83.	Superfood Chocolate-Berry Pudding	191
84.	Fig & Date Coconut Rolls	193
85.	Blissful Matcha-Pistachio Balls	194
86.	Savory Coconut Milk & Herb Whole Grain Crackers	196
87.	Crunchy Veggie Chips	198
88.	Strawberry Sorbet	199
89.	Dairy-Free Chocolate Mousse	200
90.	Steamed Broccoli and Kalamata Olives	202

91.	Sesame Carrots	204
92.	Minty-dill Beets	206
93.	Sautéed Kale with Citrus Sauce	208
94.	Spicy Frozen Orange Slices	210
95.	Tasty Fruity Salad	211
96.	Healthy Iced Green Tea	212
97.	Healthy Green Tea Latte	214
98.	Orange Mint Spritzer	215
99.	Chunky monkey smoothie with chia	216
100.	Green monster smoothie	217
101.	Peachy Coconut Smoothie	218
102.	Banana Pistachio Coconut Smoothie	218
103.	Carrot Cake Smoothie	219
Conclusion		220

Are Crohn's Disease, Inflammatory Bowel Disease and

Ulcerative Colitis all the same?

Inflammatory Bowel Disease

Unlike many gastrointestinal tract illnesses that are often attributed to poor hygiene and infections from viruses and bad bacteria, IBD is a condition that has thrived with the rise of urbanization and ever improving hygiene that has been significant from the 20th century. It is therefore safe to say that IBD is very common in developed countries. One of the main reasons for this is the lack of or reduction of germ resistance, similar to other allergic and autoimmune conditions.

For people suffering from IBD, their immune systems confuse food, the good bacteria and other substances in the gastrointestinal tract for potentially harmful foreign substances and thus reacts by dispatching the body's soldiers (white blood cells) into the lining of the bowels. This inevitable results in inflammation that develops into chronic inflammation.

Inflammatory Bowel Disease is a condition that can strike both children and adults and it's commonly diagnosed in individuals before they turn 30. It is a condition that in most cases has no cure and treatment involves managing symptoms with the main aim being remission.

For most people with IBD, it is a condition that they have to endure for the rest of their lives with alternating periods of minor and severe flare-ups and remission. With modern advances in medicine and a better understanding of nutrition and how to manage IBD, persons suffering from IBD are now able to live productive and normal lives.

Crohn's Disease

Crohn's disease has the ability to affect any part of your digestive tract starting from your mouth all the way to the anus. However, it is most commonly found in the last part of the small bowel (small intestines) and the start of the large bowel (colon).

The most common Crohn's Disease symptoms include:

- Abdominal pain
- Malnutrition
- Chronic diarrhea
- Blood-stained stool
- Constipation
- Fever
- Skin conditions such as dryness
- Weight loss
- Fatigue
- Fistula
- Joint pain

An important point to note about Crohn's disease is that it is not limited to the gastrointestinal tract. It can also affect the liver, eyes, joints and skin.

Patients with Crohn's disease usually experience worsened symptoms after taking a meal. For this reason they tend to avoid food as much as possible and that's why they tend to experience massive weight loss.

Crohn's disease can lead to intestinal blockages from repeated or chronic swelling and scarring of tissue. Ulcers in the intestinal walls if not addressed can also result in fistulas, which are tracts that form from severe sore. Patients suffering from Crohn's disease are at a higher risk of getting colon cancer and as such it is important that they have regular colonoscopies.

Ulcerative Colitis

Ulcerative colitis is a condition that affects the large intestines (colon). It mostly affects the top layers of the colon and its common symptoms include:

- Blood-stained stool
- Very loose stool
- Malnutrition
- Severe abdominal pain
- Loss of appetite
- Urgent need to make a bowel movement
- Weight loss
- Fatigue

Is it Crohn's Disease or Lactose Intolerance?

As we've already established, Crohn's Disease is a form of chronic inflammatory bowel disease that is distinguished by chronic inflammation of the gastrointestinal tract. When untreated, it can progress to serious conditions such as ulcers and fistulas. Crohn's disease symptoms are very similar to those of lactose intolerance and it's very easy for someone who has lactose intolerance to assume that the symptoms they are experiencing are those of lactose intolerance and not Crohn's disease.

To have a better understanding of how to tell lactose intolerance apart from Crohn's disease, it is important that we have a brief look into lactose intolerance.

Lactose intolerance, as the name suggests, occurs when a person is not able to synthesize enough lactase – an enzyme that is used to digest lactose, a sugar that is found in dairy. Lactase is found in the small intestines and when not enough of it is produced, it causes a lot of digestive discomfort after the consumption of dairy products. Common symptoms of lactose intolerance include:

- Sever bloating
- Diarrhea
- Abdominal pain
- Gas

Since these symptoms are similar to those of Crohn's disease, it is very possible for someone to assume they have lactose intolerance when they actually have Crohn's disease and vice versa.

Differences between Crohn's disease and Lactose Intolerance

Abdominal pain, bloating and diarrhea often accompany both lactose intolerance and Crohn's disease. However, in the case of Crohn's disease, there may be mucus or blood in stool which is not common in lactose intolerance.

Other major symptoms of Crohn's disease that are not found in lactose intolerance include:

- Fatigue
- Rapid weight loss
- Loss of appetite
- Anemia
- Fever

While lactose intolerance occurs every time a person takes dairy, Crohn's disease can go into remission for days, weeks or months at a time with very few or no symptoms at all.

Crohn's Disease Explained

Crohn's Disease is a form of Inflammatory Bowel Disease that according to the Crohn's & Colitis Foundation (CCF) affects as many as 780,000 people in America alone. This disease can affect any part of the gastrointestinal tract but it mostly affects the small and large intestines.

Here are key things you need to understand about Crohn's disease.

a. Crohn's disease has flare-up and remission phases

The symptoms that are associated with Crohn's disease, mostly associated with the inflammation of the GI tract, are at their most severe during a flare-up. When in a remission phase, Crohn's patients feel pretty normal and patients sometimes mistakenly think that they are cured and can deviate from a Crohn's disease friendly diet that again leads to a flare-up.

During a flare-up, the most common symptoms are:

- Severe abdominal pain especially right after a meal
- Blood-stained stool
- Very painful bowel movement
- Diarrhea
- Anemia
- Extreme fatigue

It's also very possible for Crohn's disease to manifest in other ways that are not typical to Chronic Inflammatory Bowel Disease such as eye inflammation and redness, joint pains and skin lesions.

b. The number of people diagnosed with Crohn's Disease increases every year

As earlier mentioned, there are 780,000 Americans diagnosed with Crohn's disease according to the Crohn's & Colitis Foundation. Diseases that are of an immune-mediated nature such as Inflammatory Bowel Diseases and Crohn's Disease in particular has been increasing steadily especially in industrialized countries.

Crohn's disease affects both men and women and symptoms can be seen at any age though it mostly manifests in teenagers and young adults of 15 to 35 years.

c. There is no known cause of Crohn's disease yet

Researchers are yet to clearly identify the primary cause of Crohn's disease. Most scientists however believe that Crohn's disease occurs as a result of a combination of a couple of factors. These include an intersection of three things, namely:

- An erratic immune system that turns on its own gastrointestinal tissue
- Genetic and/ or hereditary factors
- Environmental causes such as pollution, abuse of antibiotics, medication, infections and diet

However, more research is still underway to determine the root cause of this disease and this will play an important role in determining the best way to treat it.

d. The family tree could play a role

People with a family history Crohn's disease or Irritable Bowel Disorder have a higher risk of developing Crohn's disease or other type of Inflammatory Bowel Disease. It is however important to point out that most people who are being diagnosed with Crohn's disease do not have a family history of any form of Inflammatory Bowel Disease.

This is the reason why researchers and scientists are more inclined to believing that environmental factors plays a major role in causing Crohn's disease.

e. You can't cause Crohn's disease on yourself

While researchers and doctors are yet to specifically identify the cause of Crohn's disease, they know that it is not possible for a person to cause Crohn's disease on themselves.

f. Smoking worsens the symptoms of Crohn's disease

There is a pollution aspect of smoking that is linked to Crohn's disease. This means that smoking not only has the ability to make the symptoms of Crohn's disease more severe and more frequent, it can also significantly increase your chances of developing the disease in the first place.

According to the University of Florida, Dr. Akram, a surgeon at the university says that smoking increases flare-up occurrences by 34 percent.

g. There are many options when it comes to treating Crohn's disease.

Crohn's disease presents itself in a myriad of ways from one person to another. The number of flare-ups and remissions one person goes through are not necessarily going to be the same to another person's. For this reason, treatments are often customized to the symptoms one exhibits and also the severity of the symptoms presented.

There are a number of medical therapies that are used to treat Crohn's disease and these include the use of steroids, immunosuppresives and biologics. Other forms of treatment that are currently under research include using diet variations, probiotics, antibiotics and prebiotics to manipulate the gut bacteria. A fecal microbiota transplant is also being studied to determine its level of effectiveness. So far, the studies that have been conducted are showing promise in the treatment of Ulcerative Colitis, another type of Inflammatory Bowel Disease.

The goal of the available treatments and those that are still being researched is to target he parts of the immune function that trigger increased inflammation leading to debilitating symptoms.

In our guide, we are going to be exploring natural ways of treating Crohn's disease that help calm down flare-ups and increase the remission period for as long as possible.

h. Surgery is possible, but it's rarely a cure

There is a chance that a person suffering from Crohn's disease will undergo surgery at one point in their life, usually when medication is not enough to keep the symptoms under control. For example if there are obstructions as a result of chronic inflammation that leads to scarring. In such instances, surgery may be used to take out the severely affected parts of the GI but this is not a cure for Crohn's disease. If all other measures are thrown out the window, the symptoms continue and can lead to an obstruction at another point of the GI tract.

i. Early diagnosis will lead to effective treatment

The sooner a person is diagnosed with Crohn's disease, the higher the chances of that person getting effective treatment that will give them a high quality of life. It is important that you are able to identify a highly qualified and reputable gastroenterologist to help diagnose and guide you on the best way forward.

j. Crohn's disease often goes for a long time before being diagnosed

The availability of over the counter drugs has been a blessing and a curse in equal measures. A blessing in the sense that it is now possible for people to address health concerns such as allergies and body aches that can be very uncomfortable before seeking qualified medical assistance. A curse in the sense that most people after attaining temporary reprieve from the drugs acquired over the counter, they hardly go to the hospital to find out what was the root cause of the problem they were trying to treat.

We have become so used to the band aid approach that by the time we need to go to hospital, the problem has become so severe that drastic medical measures often have to be taken.

If you have been experiencing chronic diarrhea or abdominal pains or other persistent symptoms that we highlighted earlier such as blood in your stool, it is important that you seek the help of a gastroenterologist, share your concerns and do a couple of tests. Look at it this way, if you don't have Crohn's disease or any other form of Inflammatory Bowel Disease, then you go home with a clean bill of health. If on the other hand you are diagnosed with Crohn's Disease, you are able to catch it early and embark on a form of treatment that will take away the discomfort and pain and help you live a happy, healthy and high quality life.

k. Crohn's disease has a life-changing impact on a person.

In most cases, Crohn's disease starts when a person is very young and will stay with them for the rest of their life. This has a chance of taking a toll on even the strongest person because it means that you have to always be in high alert in terms of what you are eating, being mindful of your environment and taking stock of how your body is feeling every single day to keep tabs on whether you are having a flare-up or are in remission.

Additionally, you have to create time to keep up with medical checkups and procedure. It is important to check on your mental health on a regular basis. Why, when we are talking about a gastrointestinal problem, you may ask?

Well, picture this. You have been diagnosed with Crohn's disease after a very painful set of symptoms. You still haven't wrapped your mind around they types of food you should and shouldn't do; the amount of time you need to set aside to go see your doctor to check your progress and can't believe that this is now going to be your routine for the rest of your life.

The mere thought of going to the bathroom gives you anxiety because you don't know if you are going to see blood, if you have been on remission. And if you are in the middle of a flare-up, you don't want to deal with the pain that comes with going to the loo. Now, let's talk about being intimate. You are afraid of letting someone get close to you because you don't know if you are going to have an oops moment in the middle of an intimate moment.

Just the thought of these can give you severe anxiety and you may even develop an eating disorder which will again affect your symptoms. And so it can easily take a toll on your mental health.

We are later in the book going to be looking at how to ensure you have mind, body and spiritual health to help you live the high quality life that you deserve even as a person with Crohn's disease.

l. Support from others goes a long way.

If you or someone you know has been diagnosed with Crohn's disease, it's very important to seek or provide emotional support. You can ask your doctor to link you up with a Crohn's disease support group or you can provide support by asking to help do grocery shopping. On a bad day, something as simple as a hug goes a long way. Be mindful of your behavior around someone with Crohn's disease. For example, don't light up a cigarette because this count worsen their symptoms. Asking how you can help can also help you provide the exact amount of help that is needed. If you are the one suffering from Crohn's disease, don't be afraid to ask for help. You will be surprised by how much the people who love you are willing to go out of their way just to see be comfortable.

m. Crohn's Disease can be controlled.

The mere thought of having to live with a disease for the rest of your life can sound like the last nail on the coffin. However, with advancements in medicine and the understanding of what different foods can do for your body has made Crohn's disease quite manageable. With the help of your doctor, especially with early diagnosis, you can come up with a plan that helps manage and reduce symptoms.

Incorporating a healthy diet, fitness and meditation will also help your body find balance and operate more optimally thus keeping you in remission.

Crohn's Disease and the Stress Connection

A Body Weighed Down By Stress

How do our bodies cope with stress?

Chronic stress can wreak havoc on both mind and body. While threats from wild animals and aggressors are rarely a part of our life today, it doesn't mean that we are stress-free in today's society. We face a number of highly stressful demands each day. Health, family, work, and financial worries can easily take their toll and lead our bodies to identify these issues as a threat to our well-being. When faced with what our bodies perceive to be a dangerous or harmful situation that threatens our survival, our brains' physiological reaction is fight-or-flight. When this happens, the sympathetic nervous system stimulates the adrenal glands, which then triggers the release of catecholamines. These include adrenaline, cortisol, noradrenaline, and adrenaline.

Adrenaline

Adrenaline raises blood pressure, increases heart rate, and massively increases energy levels. It is a hormone that gets released from the adrenal glands, and along with noradrenaline, it prepares us for fight-or-flight mode.

Cortisol

Cortisol curbs non-essential or detrimental functions during a fight-or-flight situation. Cortisol alters the body's immune system responses and suppresses both the reproductive and digestive systems, and growth processes. It is Mother Nature's alarm system and communicates with the regions of the brain responsible for controlling motivation, mood, and fear. Under stressful conditions and to increase energy levels, cortisol provides our bodies with glucose. It does this by tapping into the protein stores via gluconeogenesis in the liver.

This is usually experienced as suppressed appetite and sometimes as pain in the gut.

Noradrenaline

During times of stress, noradrenaline mobilizes the body and brain, preparing it for action. When your body faces a potentially threatening occurrence, it will automatically assess how best to survive the event. Your body's immune function at this point goes on overdrive and it can even identify certain foods as being intrusive which can be a huge problem for people with Crohn's disease.

A Deeper Look at Inflammation

Inflammation has been misunderstood for the longest of time, especially seeing that it is associated with almost all chronic illnesses. However, it is important that you understand that not all inflammation spells doom for your life. Inflammation is a primal bodily response to anything considered to be a threat to your survival and existence.

Your immune system prompts inflammation when threatened by toxins, allergens, pathogens, irritants, or tissue trauma. Inflammation will then either repair damaged tissue or launch an attack of any foreign intruders, allowing your body to heal as fast as possible.

To get a truer picture of this phenomenon. If your body were without its in-built immune system, it would take less than a day for dangerous foreign bodies to attack and ultimately destroy your cells.

So if inflammation is a healthy bodily reaction, where does the problem come from?

Over time, an unhealthy lifestyle consisting of a diet of processed foods and a lack of exercise can lead to an immune system that is sluggish and that doesn't perform its duties properly. It can thus veer off course and trigger a reactive inflammatory response even when your body isn't in need of one.

As time goes on, the immune system will lose its ability to differentiate between true and false intruders. The body's immune system will then strike its organs, tissues, and cells. When this continually happens, the body gets stripped of its ability to rejuvenate, and you are likely to be diagnosed with an autoimmune disease such as Crohn's disease. For this reason, it is necessary to distinguish between healthy inflammation and unhealthy inflammation.

Acute (Healthy) Inflammation

As we have pointed out thus far, inflammation is a response that our bodies initiate to survive. Acute inflammation is triggered when your brain identifies the need for your body to heal itself from foreign intruders or tissue damage quickly.

A prime example of this is vomiting after food poisoning, whereby your body rids itself of the food you ate as quickly as possible. Doing this is a sign that your body is working hard to heal you, and once your immune system has done its job, you will notice the feeling of nausea subsiding.

Chronic (Unhealthy) inflammation

The major difference between acute inflammation and chronic inflammation is that the latter doesn't happen immediately after tissue damage or foreign intrusion. It can take anywhere from days to months or even years.

Chronic inflammation is not healing. It often leads to devastating tissue damage and serious chronic illnesses, and it is the type of inflammation that should concern us most.

Leaky Gut Syndrome

Inflammation is a precursor or catalyst to Leaky Gut Syndrome. The inner part of your gut is lined with a layer of cells that form the mucosal barrier. Nutrients are absorbed via this barrier. It also keeps germs, toxins, and large food particles from seeping into the bloodstream.

An inadequate diet can lead to an excess of yeast and toxin build up in the gut. As the body attempts to fight these toxins and waste, it becomes less effective and develops sores hat progress to holes or open ulcers that food bits can seep into the bloodstream, hence the term leaky gut.

A leaky gut then allows these toxins, germs, and undigested food particles to leak into the bloodstream, triggering a set of inflammatory responses. This can lead to food allergies, Crohn's disease, chronic fatigue, eczema, asthma, lupus, multiple sclerosis, and more.

Leaky Gut Syndrome is just one of the diseases caused by inflammation. But the same principles apply when the immune function's need to protect the body is the sole reason for causing sickness. The cause is its failure to keep pace with the attack by foreign bodies, regardless of whether they are real or caused by stress.

Causes of Chronic Inflammation

The majority of autoimmune diseases are rooted in digestive issues as a result of chronic inflammation. These we can trace to processed foods, allergens, toxins, infection, and stress. It's not all doom and gloom, though. The leading cause of chronic inflammation is a combination of a diet consisting of over-processed foods and a sedentary lifestyle. Both of which we can easily change.

Starting the Healing Process

Inflammation and Stress Explained

Inflammation is the most common stress response. It can help prevent wound infection, drive toxins out of the body, and induce diarrhea to eliminate pathogens from your gut. It may even cause pain and swelling to an injured body part to render it painful. It does this with the aim of promoting rest and accelerate healing on the particular part.

In the case of digestive stress, where inflammation is caused by continued stress and, in particular, digestive inflammation from a poor diet, or continued intake of food that your body is 'allergic' to such as gluten, the brain's communication with the adrenal nodes can become distorted.

Your body's responses are brain-initiated, survival tactics, and, in the short term, are extremely useful. Unfortunately, however, if you are subjected continually to fight-or-flight situations, your body's ability to respond to imminent danger gets worn down. When this happens, your brain's effort to spark response transforms into debilitating stress. You will then experience a sick gut, irritability and fatigue, to name but a few.

Chronic inflammation may also occur due to obesity, non-healing infections, and your body's immune system attacking normal body tissues. When this condition persists, it creeps up to your vital organs. In which case, your digestive system may develop sores and lead to painful inflamed bowel diseases such as Crohn's disease.

Your kidneys may be unable to filter out toxins. Your liver may become so overwhelmed with the processes of synthesizing fat that it begins to store fat, leading to fatty liver disease. When this happens, your body is then not able to optimally absorb nutrients from the food you eat, blood vessels become thinner meaning blood is no longer being pumped efficiently, leading to chronic illnesses.

In extreme cases, your DNA may become compromised. For example, a person who has Crohn's disease or ulcerative colitis may be at a greater risk of contracting colorectal cancer.

It is therefore of utmost importance that you pay attention to what we eat and listen to what our bodies are trying to communicate. Eliminate foods that will fail to spark an immune response and instead choose ones that will nourish and energize your body. Remember, you are what you eat!

Effective Ways of Healing Crohn's Disease

Symptoms

So far we have established that your immune function plays a major role in triggering Crohn's disease.

Life is a challenge, but it can become a daily uphill struggle when you are constantly weighed down by pain especially every time you eat. One of the main culprits of dwindling energy levels is the food we eat, let alone your body not being able to utilize it.

Pre-prepared meals, fast, and processed foods are often high in fat, sugar, and salt, and many contain empty calories. They offer very little nutritional value and result in us feeling hungry and lacking in energy.

Some commercially produced foods contain not only artificial sweeteners and colorings but also Trans fats.

It is these that compromise our digestive system especially if you have an overly sensitive immune function as it will interpret these as harmful substances.

Poor nutrition can also cause chronic fatigue as our major organs, including the liver, heart, and brain, become starved of the fuel they need to function. Chronic fatigue is your body's cry for help and a warning sign that it is time to enjoy a healthy, well-balanced diet and lifestyle.

The key in healing your gut is in proper medical testing to confirm whether the pain, discomfort, bloating, diarrhea, fever and other symptoms that you have been experiencing are as a result of Crohn's disease. Once you are sure of the answer, there are many ways in which you can heal your gut and go back to your energetic, happier and vibrant self.

Here are some of the ways of healing your gut:

1. Eliminate as many ways of triggering an immune response as possible

Start by running an audit of your lifestyle dating back to when you started experience the symptoms of Crohn's disease. The best place to start with is your diet. Eliminate all processed foods and instead focus on fresh, healthy, natural and unprocessed foods, preferably organic.

You can also test to find out whether you are allergic to gluten as this can result in inflammation and consequently an inflamed gut

Supporting your body's natural detoxification process will also help your gastrointestinal tract. Avoid foods and anything you get in contact with that's doused with chemicals. You can start growing a few veggies organically in your kitchen garden or buying organic food at farmers' markets.

Stress is another contributor to inflammation. Change your attitude towards life and surround yourself with positive energy and positive people.

2. Engage in regular physical activity

Exercising on a regular basis boosts tissue sensitivity and an overally healthy body. Do exercises that will get your heart pumping and your body sweating. After working up a healthy sweat you can relax in a sauna and help your body get rid of excess toxins through sweating, every once in a while. Hydrating well after a workout will also do the trick. This will help in eliminating toxins that goes a long way in boosting the health of your gut.

3. Eliminate your symptoms nutritionally

Healing for your gut depends on a healthy and balanced nutrition. You can boost the secretion of digestive enzymes and the multiplication of gut healthy bacteria by taking natural and unprocessed foods. Gut –healthy foods include probiotic rich foods such as yogurt, kombucha; omega-3 fat high foods such as wild caught fish especially salmon and sardines, dark leafy greens including dandelions and mustard and other whole foods.

The secret is to avoid foods that can negatively impact on your gut such as gluten and processed foods.

4. Drink plenty of water

Your body needs optimum hydration to reduce inflammation in your body that is caused by toxin buildup. For a single pound of body weight, you should drink 0.5 to 1 ounce of water each day. For example, if you weigh 140 pounds, you should be drinking between 70-140 ounces (approximately 10 cups) of water every day. Doing this is essential to reducing the symptoms of Crohn's disease.

5. Reduce alcohol consumption and stop smoking

Most of us enjoy a glass of our favorite alcoholic drink every now and then, sometimes more than we should, but we need to be aware of its effect on our overall gastrointestinal health.

The good bacteria in our guts help us to process alcohol. For this reason, tolerance to alcohol can vary from person to person. If your body's gut flora is compromised, it will affect how well it can detoxify the alcohol.

Drink too much, there is a higher chance that the process of secreting enzymes and juices is going to be affected thus affecting the whole digestive process meaning it becomes increasingly difficult for the body to absorb the nutrients from the food ingested.

Let alone the fact that food that is only partially processed can lead to gas, uncomfortable bloating, and loose bowel movements, symptoms that can exacerbate Crohn's disease.

Excessive consumption of alcohol can also trigger inflammation in the gut. This condition can then lead to your gut lining, becoming more permeable, and allowing particles of food to cross the lining and enter the bloodstream. Sometimes this can then lead to new food intolerances and very painful Crohn's disease flare-ups.

Cigarette smoking is a complete no – no as it has been linked to triggering Crohn's disease. If you been enjoying a calm remission phase, smoking could very easily take you down the rabbit hole of unimaginable pain of discomfort that comes with the flare-up phase.

When you do feel like the occasional alcoholic drink, then opt for a small glass of red wine, preferably dry or semi-sweet. Red wine contains polyphenols, such as resveratrol found in red grape skin, eucalyptus, nuts, berries, and fir leaves. These micronutrients are believed to have beneficial properties that act as fuel for microbes living inside the intestines.

6. Make naturally occurring super foods an integral part of your diet

Foods that are rich in probiotics and prebiotics can aid your digestive function. These foods include natural yogurt, kombucha, kimchi, tempeh, miso, saltwater-brined pickles, and sauerkraut. They each contain friendly bacteria that will help fight off bad bacteria to reduce inflammation.

Omega-3 fats are also essential in boosting immunity. These include oily fish such as salmon, herrings, sardines, as well as seeds such as chia, sunflower, and pumpkin seeds.

What's more, flavor food with fresh herbs and spices. Cayenne pepper, garlic, ginger, and turmeric all have potent anti-inflammatory benefits. Dark-colored berries are also rich in anti-inflammatories, such as anthocyanins, that fight off free radicals. These molecules with unpaired electrons rob other cells of electrons, causing damage and contributing to some diseases.

7. Cut out processed sugar

Processed sugars only feed the bad bacteria in our gut and cause insulin spikes. Go for natural sweeteners such as raw honey, maple syrup and fruit. An important point to note is that just because it is natural doesn't mean you can meat as much as you possibly want.

Take sugar sparingly to avoid flare-ups.

8. Reduce your intake of take-out

Most take-out contains a lot of extra sugar, salt, oil, and of course, excess calories.

With Crohn's disease, it is extremely important that you eliminate processed sugar, carbs, artificial sweeteners, Trans fats, and other over-processed foods from your body. They will increase your caloric intake, trigger inflammation, and are of very little nutritional benefit.

9. Recipes for Crohn's disease

Later on in the book, check out our simple, tasty and healing collection of recipes. Here, you will find mouthwateringly good meals, snacks, and drinks that are anything but boring or flare-up triggering!

10. Take food supplements (if necessary)

While it's always advisable to get all the nutrition you need from natural food, you may find yourself in a situation that requires you to take certain food supplements especially if you are allergic to a particular food.

With Crohn's disease, it is very possible that a certain type of food could induce a flare-up and your doctor could therefore advise that you take specific supplements. However, only do this under your doctor's advisement.

11. Go for medical checkup

Crohn's disease is not the easiest ailment to identify and the best thing you can do for yourself is to go see your doctor, describe all your symptoms and they'll advise you on the tests to take. After the results come out, your doctor will advise you on the best course of action depending on whether you tested positive or negative for Crohn's disease.

12. A healthy sleep pattern

Aim for around 6-8 hours of uninterrupted sleep. Doing this will help your body relax. It will also allow you to recover from the day's stresses and recharge your batteries for the next day.

Time spent asleep is an excellent investment in your health, so don't be tempted to get by on just a few hours of shut-eye each night. Lack of sleep can have an adverse effect on recovery times after sickness.

.Avoid watching TV, working on your computer, or looking at your phone or tablet at least an hour before you head to bed. Instead, read a book or take 10-15 minutes to reflect on your day. Alternatively, listen to soothing music or sounds that will help you drift off into a relaxing sleep.

13. Meditation and Reflection

When it comes to reducing inflammation, a healthy mind is as essential as a healthy body. Aim to maintain a clear and untroubled mind as much as possible. The human brain is the smartest computer ever made and can detect even the smallest hint of an issue or problem. You can avoid stressful situations by taking some time out each day to reflect and meditate on your life, its issues, and the solutions you need to implement.

You may also like to consider taking up yoga. Certain poses can help detox the body, aid digestion, and relieve stress to naturally reduce chronic inflammation.

Benefits of Healing Your Gut

Great health is the perfect gift you can get yourself and healing your gut will make you rediscover life in a way you never thought possible. Some of the benefits you are sure to see include:

- Increased energy

Forget about breakfast coffee. A perfectly working gut will make you feel superb!

- Healthy weight

Severe weight loss is one of the most annoying side effects of Crohn's disease. Healing your gut and continuing with a healthy diet and regular exercise regimen will help you gain healthy weight and keep you strong.

- Clarity of mind

When everything in your body is working perfectly, you won't have to fight yourself to go through a work day with several coffees.

- Sleep like an angel

Forget about the days of insomnia because of the pain. With a healed gut, you are going to feel amazing and you will always sleep the night through and have loads of energy on waking up.

- The fountain of youth

You will feel forever young with an added spring to your step thanks to a healed gut as you can count on the nutrients from the food you eat to be fully absorbed into your bloodstream and to be transported to the organs.

Crohn's Disease Eating Recap

To recap, here is a brief summary of what to eat:

- **Choose Green Always**

Green vegetables are vitamin, protein, and fiber-rich. Fiber is really good for digestion and can help your body eliminate toxins. It does this by binding to toxins and eliminating them from the body through waste.

- **Color and Texture**

Halt junk food cravings by keeping your food choices exciting and varied. Experiment with different colored and textured ingredients to help banish meal-time boredom.

- **Fresh is Life**

Choose only fresh foods. If an item is canned or boxed, eliminate it from your eating plan. They do not contain the same nutritional benefits. Instead of buying canned or powdered chicken broth, make your own over the weekend and use it for your weekday cooking and reserve the meat for sandwiches and other chicken dinners.

Do this, and you will see a noticeable improvement in your digestion, skin, and weight.

- **Spice your World**

Are you confused about the difference between fresh herbs and spices? You're not alone! Whether fresh or dry, herbs are the plant leaves, while spices are every other part, including roots, flowers, stems, berries, and seeds. Herbs and spices can elevate daily dishes and add flavor to mealtimes. What's more, they pack a powerful punch when it comes to gut health. They play a leading role in helping to break down the food our bodies can't digest. For example, when cooked into food, cardamom is believed to balance mucus, gas, and bloating in both the small intestine and stomach.

Ginger helps in bloating and constipation. Basil can reduce gas and stomach cramping, and bay leaves can help to soothe irritable bowel syndrome.

If you are looking at new ways to use herbs and spices in your everyday cooking, then check out our Recipes for Success section at the end of this book!

Part Two: CHRON'S-TREATMENT MEAL PLAN & RECIPES

Please make sure when you do the meal plan, that the calorie intake will be sufficient for your body.

30-DAY CHRON'S DIET MEAL PLAN

Day	Breakfast	AM SNACK	Lunch	PM SNACK	Dinner
DAY 1	Gut-Healing Ginger Pineapple Juice	1 Glass Juice for Gut Health	Gut Healing Soup with Mashed Potatoes	1 Glass Orange & Aloe Vera Juice	Grilled Chicken with Fresh Herb Marinade
DAY 2	Chia Seed & Peanut Butter Protein Pudding	Delicious Mashed Lime Peas	Protein Chicken Curry with Coconut Rice	1 Glass Stomach Soothing Juice	Salmon Served with Mashed Potatoes

DAY 3	Healthy Avocado & Berry Acai Smoothie	1 Glass Healthy Iced Green Tea	Spinach & Turkey Soup Pasta	Gut Friendly Smoothie	Super Tasty Mushroom Marinara with Pasta
DAY 4	Ginger and Red Onion Pancakes	Delicious Humus	Delicious Low Carb Chicken Curry with Steamed White Rice	1 Cup Detoxifying Turmeric Tea	Creamy Citrus Salmon Baked in Coconut Milk
DAY 5	Gut-Healing Chocolate Breakfast Shake	1 Glass Green Fruit Drink	Zucchini & Mushroom Soup with Mashed Potatoes	Sautéed Kale with Citrus Sauce	Curried Prawns with White Bread
DAY 6	Coconut Yogurt Peanut Butter Parfait	Easy and Tasty Pumpkin Muffin in a Cup	Grilled Shiitake Mushrooms	1 Glass Orange Mint Spritzer	Grilled Beef & White Rice
DAY 7	Healthy Whole Food Breakfast Smoothie	Superfood Chocolate-Berry Pudding	Italian Fish Stew with Yummy Mashed Potatoes	1 Glass Healthy Green Tea Latte	Tilapia with Mushroom Sauce

DAY 8	Spring Onion & Salmon Frittata	1 Glass Chunky monkey smoothie with chia	Spinach & Turkey Soup with Steamed White Rice	Dairy-Free Chocolate Mousse	Grilled Chicken with Fresh Herb Marinade
DAY 9	Healthy Berry Breakfast Shake	Green Peanut Butter Smoothie	Healthy Protein-Packed Fish Tikka Curry with Pasta	1 Glass Green monster smoothie	White Fish & Coconut Rice
DAY 10	Gut-Healing Smoothie	1 Glass Stomach Soothing Juice	Lean Steak & Mung Cleansing Soup with Mashed Potatoes	Delicious Mashed Lime Peas	Super Tasty Mushroom Marinara with Pasta
DAY 11	Superfood Breakfast Bowl	Steamed Broccoli and Kalamata Olives	Lean Steak & Veggie in Coconut Curry Sauce with Steamed White Rice	1 Glass Banana Pistachio Coconut Smoothie	Tasty Coconut Cod

DAY 12	Healthy Coconut Pancakes	1 Glass Peachy Coconut Smoothie	Grilled Shiitake Mushrooms	1 Glass Carrot Cake Smoothie	Grilled Chicken with Fresh Herb Marinade
DAY 13	Healing Green Smoothie	Carrot Cake Smoothie	Shrimp & Pineapple Curry	1 Glass Orange Mint Spritzer	Creamy Citrus Salmon Baked in Coconut Milk
DAY 14	Turmeric Almond Milk & Berry Shake	1 Glass Orange & Aloe Vera Juice	Spinach & Turkey Soup with Pasta	Raw Banana Mash Snack	Salmon Served with Mashed Potatoes
DAY 15	Scrambled Eggs & Grilled Salmon with Avocado	1 Glass Healthy Iced Green Tea	Lettuce Avocado & Egg Salad Wraps	Crunchy Veggie Chips	Sweet Potato & Herbed Chicken Casserole

DAY 16	Ginger Berry Anti-Inflammatory Smoothie	Dairy-Free Chocolate Mousse	Healthy Savory Beef Stew	1 Glass Chunky monkey smoothie with chia	Super Tasty Mushroom Marinara with Pasta
DAY 17	Healthy Breakfast Casserole	1 Glass Peachy Coconut Smoothie	Healthy Beef Lettuce Wraps	Sesame Carrots	Grilled Steak Salad with Red Onion, Orange & Avocado
DAY 18	Ginger Detox Smoothie	Strawberry Sorbet	Tasty Bean Soup with Tortilla Chips	1 Glass Healthy Green Tea Latte	Stir Fried Beef with Veggies
DAY 19	Cheesy Red Onion Omelet	1 Glass Green Peanut Butter Smoothie	Healthy Savory Beef Stew with Avocado	Blissful Matcha-Pistachio Balls	White Fish & Coconut Rice
DAY 20	Spicy Breakfast Carrot Pudding	Minty-dill Beets	Vegan Red Lentil Soup	1 Glass Juice for Gut Health	Ginger Chicken with Veggies

DAY 21	Scrambled Eggs & Grilled Salmon with Avocado	Banana Pistachio Coconut Smoothie	Sauteed Green Bean & Zucchini Bowl	1 Glass Green monster smoothie	Tasty Coconut Cod
DAY 22	Peanut Butter Chocolate Swirl Porridge	1 Glass Peachy Coconut Smoothie	Protein Chicken Curry with Coconut Rice	Tasty Fruity Salad	Curried Prawns with White Bread
DAY 23	Salmon Omelet	Spicy Frozen Orange Slices	Mango & Grilled Steak Salad w/ Buttermilk-Avocado Buttermilk Dressing	1 Glass Healthy Iced Green Tea	Lemon BBQ Salmon
DAY 24	Mushroom & Tomato Omelet	1 Glass Carrot Cake Smoothie	Crunchy Salmon Arugula Salad	Sautéed Kale with Citrus Sauce	Grilled Chicken with Fresh Herb Marinade
DAY 25	Ginger and Red Onion Pancakes	Crunchy Veggie Chips	Chickpea Salad Wrap	1 Glass Green monster smoothie	Spiced Roast Side of Salmon

DAY 26	Turmeric Almond Milk & Berry Shake	1 Glass Chunky monkey smoothie with chia	Tasty Lime Cilantro Cauliflower Rice	Fig & Date Coconut Rolls	Chili Fried Steak with Toasted Cashews
DAY 27	Coconut Yogurt Peanut Butter Parfait	Superfood Chocolate-Berry Pudding	Lemony Squash Salad	1 Glass Stomach Soothing Juice	Super Tasty Mushroom Marinara with Pasta
DAY 28	Detox Oatmeal Porridge	Chocolaty Kamut Energy Bars	Turmeric Chickpea & Artichoke Sauté	1 Glass Orange Mint Spritzer	Hot Lemon Garlic Prawns with Rice
DAY 29	Shrimp & Avocado Omelet	1 Glass Healthy Green Tea Latte	Lunch Salad with Lemony Dressing	Savory Coconut Milk & Herb Whole Grain Crackers	Tilapia with Mushroom Sauce
DAY 30	Chai-Cashew Latte Oatmeal	Blissful Matcha-Pistachio Balls	Protein Chicken Curry with Coconut Rice	1 Glass Juice for Gut Health	Sweet Potato & Herbed Chicken Casserole

CHRON'S DIET BREAKFAST RECIPES

1. Gut-Healing Chocolate Breakfast Shake

Yield: 1 Serving

Total Time: 5 Minutes

Prep Time: 5 Minutes

Cook Time: N/A

Ingredients

- ¼ avocado
- 1 ripe banana
- 1 cup almond milk
- 2 tablespoons cacao powder
- 1 teaspoon maca powder
- 3 tablespoons protein powder

Directions

Combine all ingredients in a blender and blend until very smooth. Enjoy!

2. Chia Seed & Peanut Butter Protein Pudding

Yield: 1 Serving

Total Time: 5 Minutes

Prep Time: 5 Minutes

Cook Time: N/A

Ingredients
- 20g natural peanut butter
- 200g unsweetened almond milk
- 1/2 banana
- 10g chia seeds
- 10g flaxseeds
- 25g vanilla protein powder

Directions
In a blender, blend together peanut butter, milk and banana until very smooth; transfer to a serving bowl and stir in chia seeds and flaxseeds. Chill, covered, for at least 4 hours. When ready, stir and serve.

Nutritional Information Per Serving:
Calories: 407; Total Fat: 20.7; Carbs: 28.9 g; Dietary Fiber: 9.7 g; Sugars: 9.4; Protein: 28.9 g; Cholesterol: 52 mg; Sodium: 192 mg

3. Healthy Avocado & Berry Acai Smoothie

Yield: 2 Servings

Total Time: 10 Minutes

Prep Time: 10 Minutes

Cook Time: N/A

Ingredients
- 1/2 avocado
- ½ cup blackberries
- ½ cup strawberries
- ½ cup raspberries
- 1 heaped tablespoon acai powder
- 1 cup chopped kale leaves
- 1 tablespoon almond butter
- 1/2 cup almond milk

Directions
In a blender, blend all ingredients until very smooth.

Nutritional Information per Serving:
Calories: 336; Total Fat: 29.9 g; Carbs: 10.6 g; Dietary Fiber: 3.2 g; Sugars: 7.8 g; Protein: 4.3 g; Cholesterol: 0 mg; Sodium: 24 mg

4. Spring Onion & Salmon Frittata

Yield: 6 servings

Total Time: 30 Minutes

Prep Time: 10 Minutes

Cook Time: 20 Minutes

Ingredients

- 2 teaspoons extra-virgin olive oil
- 6 spring onions, trimmed and chopped
- 4 large eggs
- 6 large egg whites
- ½ teaspoon finely chopped fresh tarragon
- ¼ cup water
- ½ teaspoon salt
- 2 ounces smoked salmon, sliced into small pieces
- 2 tablespoons black olive tapenade

Directions

Preheat your oven to 350°F.

Set a large ovenproof pan over medium heat; add oil and heat until hot, but not smoky. Stir in spring onions and sauté, stirring, for about 3 minutes or until tender and fragrant. In a bowl, beat together eggs, egg whites, tarragon, water, and salt; season with black pepper and pour into the pan. Arrange the salmon onto the egg mixture. Cook, stirring frequently, for about 2 minutes or until almost set; transfer to the oven and cook for about 14 minutes or until puffed and golden. Remove the frittata from the oven and transfer to a serving plate; slice and serve with tapenade.

Nutritional Information per Serving:

Calories: 186; Total Fat: 5 g; Carbs: 1 g; Dietary Fiber: trace; Protein: 10 g; Cholesterol: 143 mg; Sodium: 535 mg; Sugars: trace

5. Chai-Cashew Latte Oatmeal

Yield: 4 Servings

Total Time: 30 Minutes

Prep Time: 10 Minutes

Cook Time: 20 Minutes

Ingredients

- 2 cups coconut milk
- 4 Chai tea bags
- 2 cups unsweetened cashew milk
- 2 cups rolled oats
- ½ teaspoon cinnamon
- ¼ teaspoon cardamom
- ½ cup toasted coconut
- ½ cup cashew pieces
- 2 bananas, sliced
- ½ teaspoon sea salt

Directions

Simmer a cup of coconut milk in a small saucepan over medium heat; add the tea bags and steep for about 10 minutes.

In the meantime, simmer the remaining coconut creamer and cashew milk over medium heat and stir in oats; simmer for about 15 minutes or until thick.

Stir in strained chai cream, half of cinnamon, cardamom, and sea salt; ladle into serving bowls and top with toasted coconut, cashews, sliced banana and more cinnamon. Enjoy!

Nutritional Information per Serving:

Calories: 384 Total Fat: 15.4 g; Carbs: 54.9 g; Dietary Fiber: 7.4 g; Sugars: 11.1 g; Protein: 9.6 g; Cholesterol: 0 mg; Sodium: 322 mg

6. Gut-Healing Ginger Pineapple Juice

Yield: 1 Serving

Total Time: 5 Minutes

Prep Time: 5 Minutes

Cook Time: N/A

Ingredients

- ½ pineapple
- 1 lemon
- Fresh ginger
- Fresh turmeric
- 1 handful mint

Directions

Juice all the ingredients and pour the juice into a tall glass. Enjoy!

7. Detox Oatmeal Porridge

Yield: 4 Servings

Total Time: 12 Minutes

Prep Time: 5 Minutes

Cook Time: 7 Minutes

Ingredients
- 1 cup almond milk
- 1 cup rolled oats
- 1 cup blueberries
- 1 teaspoon coconut oil
- 3 teaspoons raw honey
- 1 peach, peeled, thinly sliced

Directions

Combine milk and oats in a small pan set over medium heat; bring to a gentle boil. Simmer for about 5 minutes, stirring frequently; transfer the mixture to a blender and add in berries, coconut oil and raw honey; blend until very smooth.

Ladle porridge into serving bowls and top each with peach slices, and raw honey. Enjoy!

Nutritional Information per Serving:

Calories: 277; Total Fat: 17 g; Carbs: 30.2 g; Dietary Fiber: 4.9 g; Sugars: 23.6 g; Protein: 4.7 g; Cholesterol: 0 mg; Sodium: 11 mg

8. Shrimp & Avocado Omelet

Yields: 1 Serving

Total Time: 40 Minutes

Prep Time: 10 Minutes

Cook Time: 30 Minutes

Ingredients

- 60g shrimp, peeled and de-veined
- 2 free-range eggs, beaten
- 1/4 medium avocado, diced
- 1 medium tomato, diced
- 10g butter
- 1/8 teaspoon pepper
- 1/4 teaspoon sea salt
- 10g freshly chopped cilantro

Directions

Cook shrimp in a skillet set over medium heat until it turns pink; chop the cooked shrimp and set aside.

In a small bowl, toss together avocado, tomato, and cilantro; season with sea salt and pepper and set aside.
In a separate bowl, beat the eggs and set aside.
Set a skillet over medium heat; add butter and heat until hot.

Add the egg to the skillet and tilt the skillet to cover the bottom. When almost cooked, add shrimp onto one side of the egg and fold in half. Cook for 1 minute more and top with the avocado-tomato mixture.

Repeat with the remaining ingredients for the second omelet.

Nutritional Information Per Serving:
Calories: 396; Total Fat: 28 g; Carbs: 11.2 g; Dietary Fiber: 5.2 g; Sugars: 4.3g; Protein: 27.1 g; Cholesterol: 475 mg; Sodium: 809 mg

9. Coconut Yogurt Peanut Butter Parfait

Ingredients

- 1 cup coconut yogurt
- 2 bananas
- 1 cup papaya chunks
- 2 smooth peanut butter

Directions

Divide coconut yogurt in two tall glasses; layer with papaya chunks and banana slices. Top with smoot peanut butter. Enjoy!

10. Healthy Whole Food Breakfast Smoothie

Yield: 4 Servings

Total Time: 10 Minutes

Prep Time: 10 Minutes

Cook Time: N/A

Ingredients:

- 1 cup frozen blueberries
- 2 teaspoons flaxseed
- 2 teaspoons chia seeds
- ½ cup nonfat Greek yogurt
- ½ cup almon milk
- 1 banana, peeled, chopped
- 1 pear, peeled

Directions

Combine all ingredients in a blender and blend until very smooth. Enjoy!

Nutrition info Per Serving:

Calories: 191; Total Fat: 3.2 g; Carbs: 30.9 g; Dietary Fiber: 4.7 g; Sugars: 18.8; Protein: 9 g; Cholesterol: 3 mg; Sodium: 52 m

11. Cheesy Red Onion Omelet

Yield: 1 Serving

Total Time: 20 Minutes

Prep Time: 10 Minutes

Cook Time: 10 Minutes

Ingredients

- 10g butter
- 2 large eggs
- 1 red onion, finely chopped
- 10g chopped parsley
- 50g cheddar cheese
- Handful rocket leaves
- Salt and pepper

Directions

Heat oil in a frying pan set over medium low heat; stir in the red onion and fry for about 5 minutes. Cook over medium heat for about 2 minutes.

Whisk the eggs well and add to the pan with the onion; evenly distribute the egg mixture and cook for about 1 minute.

Sprinkle with grated cheese and lift the sides of the omelet to allow the uncooked egg slip in the base of the frying pan. Cook to your desired doneness and sprinkle with parsley and rocket; Season with salt and pepper and roll up the omelet.

Serve right away.

Nutritional Information Per Serving
Calories: 465; Total Fat: 34.8 g; Carbs: 12.5 g; Dietary fiber: 2.8 g; Sugars: 5.8 g; Protein: 26.7 g; Cholesterol: 446 mg; Sodium: 519 mg

12. Healthy Berry Breakfast Shake

Yield: 1 to 2 Servings

Total Time: 5 Minutes

Prep Time: 5 Minutes

Cook Time: 0 Minutes

Ingredients

- ½ tbsp. ground chia seeds
- ½ tsp. vanilla extract
- 100g vanilla protein powder
- ½ cup lemon juice
- 1/2 cup almond milk
- 1 cup frozen strawberries
- 1 cup blackberries

Directions

Combine all ingredients in a blender. Blend until very smooth.
Enjoy!

Nutritional Information per Serving:
Calories: 453; Total Fat: 22.2g; Carbs: 39 g; Dietary Fiber: 6.3 g; Sugars: 17.8 g; Protein: 28.4 g; Cholesterol: 5 mg; Sodium: 137 mg

13. Ginger and Red Onion Pancakes

Yield: 4 Servings

Total Time: 26 Minutes

Prep Time: 10 Minutes

Cook Time: 16 Minutes

Ingredients

- 1 1/2 tablespoons coconut oil
- 3/4 cup coconut milk
- 8 eggs
- 1/4 cup tapioca flour
- 1/4 cup almond flour
- 100g whey protein powder
- 1 teaspoon salt
- ½ inch ginger, grated
- 1 handful cilantro, chopped
- ½ red onion, chopped

Directions
In a bowl, whisk eggs, coconut milk, tapioca flour, almond flour, and protein powder until well blended; stir in ginger, cilantro, and red onion until well combined.

Melt coconut oil in a saucepan over medium low heat; add about ¼ cup of batter and spread out on the pan. Cook for about 4 minutes per side or until golden brown.

Transfer to a plate and keep warm; repeat with the remaining batter and oil.

Serve the pancakes with freshly squeezed orange juice.

Nutritional Information per Serving:
Calories: 371; Total Fat: 28.2 g; Carbs: 20.9 g; Dietary Fiber: 2.1g; Sugars: 4.2 g; Protein: 26.9 g; Cholesterol: 330 mg; Sodium: 787 mg

14. Gut-Healing Smoothie

Yield: 2 Servings

Total Time: 5 Minutes

Prep Time: 5 Minutes

Cook Time: N/A

Ingredients:

- 2 cups almond milk
- 2 frozen bananas
- 1/2 avocado
- 2 cups spinach
- 2 cups kale
- 1 tablespoon hemp hearts
- 1/2 tablespoon chia seeds
- 1 teaspoon grated ginger
- 2 tablespoons protein powder
- 1/2 tablespoon raw honey

Directions

Combine all ingredients in a blender and blend until very smooth. Enjoy!

Nutritional Information per Serving:
Calories: 296; Total Fat: 19.2 g; Carbs: 28 g; Dietary Fiber: 4.5 g; Sugars: 13.9.1 g; Protein: 8.6 g; Cholesterol: 0 mg; Sodium: 55 mg

15.   Salmon Omelet

Yield: 1 Servings

Total Time: 20 Minutes

Prep Time: 10 Minutes

Cook Time: 10 Minutes

Ingredients

- 1 tsp. extra virgin olive oil
- 100 g sliced smoked salmon
- ½ cup chopped spring onions
- 1/2 teaspoon capers
- 2 large eggs
- 10g chopped rocket
- 1 teaspoon chopped parsley

Directions

Beat the eggs into a large bowl; stir in salmon, spring onions, rocket, capers, and chopped parsley.
Add extra virgin olive oil to a nonstick pan and heat over medium heat until hot, but not smoking; add the egg mixture and spread the mixture evenly in the pan. Lower heat and cook until the omelet is cooked through. With a spatula, roll up the omelet in half and serve hot.

Nutritional Information Per Serving

Calories: 303; Total Fat: 19 g; Carbs: 1.3 g; Dietary fiber: trace; Sugars: 1 g; Protein: 31.2 g; Cholesterol: 395 mg; Sodium: 2186 mg

16. Turmeric Almond Milk & Berry Shake

Yield: 4 Servings

Total Time: 5 Minutes

Prep Time: 5 Minutes

Cook Time: N/A

Ingredients
- ½ cup blackberries
- ½ cup strawberries
- ½ cup raspberries
- 2 cups almond milk
- 1/4 cup smooth peanut butter
- 1 teaspoon turmeric
- 1 teaspoon liquid stevia

Directions
Blend everything together until very smooth. Enjoy!

Nutritional Information per Serving:
Calories: 378; Total Fat: 35.8 g; Carbs: 5.9 g; Dietary Fiber: 7 g; Sugars: 7.8 g; Protein: 5.3 g; Cholesterol: 0 mg; Sodium: 20 mg

17. Superfood Breakfast Bowl

Yield: 3 Servings

Total Time: 5 Minutes

Prep Time: 5 Minutes

Cook Time: 5 Minutes

Ingredients:
- ½ cup strawberries
- ½ cup blackberries
- ½ cup raspberries
- ½ cup goji berries
- 2 tablespoons acai powder
- 1 teaspoon lucuma powder
- ½ cup peeled and diced mango
- 1/2 cup almond milk

Directions:
In a blender, blend all ingredients until very smooth. Enjoy!

Nutritional Information per Serving:
Calories: 413; Total Fat: 26.8 g; Carbs: 45.6 g; Dietary Fiber: 12.5 g; Sugars: 28.1 g; Protein: 4.7 g; Cholesterol: 0 mg; Sodium: 19 mg

18. Healing Green Smoothie

Yield: 6 Servings

Total Time: 5 Minutes

Prep Time: 5 Minutes

Cook Time: N/A

Ingredients

- ½ avocado
- 2 celery stalks
- 6 medium strawberries
- 1 cup chopped carrots
- 1 apple
- 3 larges leaves of kale
- 5 large leaves of romaine lettuce
- 3 cups coconut water

Directions

Combine all ingredients in a blender and blend until very smooth. Enjoy!

Nutritional Information per Serving:

Calories: 69; Total Fat: 3.4 g; Carbs: 10.2 g; Dietary Fiber: 2.8 g; Sugars: 5.1 g; Protein: 1 g; Cholesterol: 0 mg; Sodium: 21 mg

19. Scrambled Eggs & Grilled Salmon with Avocado

Yield: 2 Servings

Total Time: 25 Minutes

Prep Time: 10 Minutes

Cook Time: 15 Minutes

Ingredients

- 2 leftover grilled salmon fillets, chopped
- 2 eggs
- 1 tablespoon extra-virgin olive oil
- 1 cup diced spring onions
- 2 cloves garlic
- 1 cup pureed tomatoes
- salt and pepper
- Avocado, diced

Directions

Heat olive oil in a pan over medium heat; sauté red onions, garlic and pureed tomatoes for about 5 minutes or until tender. Beat eggs, salt, and pepper until well combined. Stir in chopped spring onions and add to the pan.

Cook for about 5 minutes or until set to your liking. Warm your leftover grilled salmon and serve with the scrambled eggs topped with avocado slices on the side.

Nutrition information per Serving:
Calories: 620; Total Fat: 45.3 g; Carbs: 19.3 g; Dietary Fiber: 10.1 g; Sugars: 5.9 g; Protein: 42.1 g; Cholesterol: 78 mg; Sodium: 122 mg

20. Herbs Omelet

Yield: 1 Serving

Ingredients
- 2 eggs
- Pinch of salt
- Pinch of salt
- 10g coconut oil
- 30g grated cheddar cheese
- 30g chopped parsley
- 30g chopped green onion
- 5g dried tarragon
- 5g finely chopped garlic

Directions

In a bowl, beat the eggs together with salt and pepper until well combined. Stir in the herbs until well combined.
Melt coconut oil a skillet set over medium heat. Pour in the egg mixture and cook until the egg is almost set. Sprinkle grated cheese over one half of the omelet; with a spatula, fold the other half of the omelet over onto the filled half. Cook for a few seconds or until the cheese is melted and egg is set. Enjoy!

Nutritional Information per Serving:
Calories: 418; Total Fat: 31.2 g; Carbs: 7.2 g; Dietary Fiber: 1.7 g; Sugars: 2.8 g; Protein: 27.5 g; Cholesterol: 409 mg; Sodium: 1176 mg

21. Ginger Berry Anti-Inflammatory Smoothie

Yield: 2 Servings

Total Time: 5 Minutes

Prep Time: 5 Minutes

Cook Time: N/A

Ingredients

- 1 cup Greek yogurt
- 1 cup frozen strawberries
- 1 cup frozen blueberries
- 1 cup celery
- 1 cup kale
- 1 cup spinach
- 2 inch piece ginger
- 3 tablespoons hemp protein powder

Directions

Combine all ingredients in a blender and blend until very smooth. Enjoy!

22. Peanut Butter Chocolate Swirl Porridge

Yield: 1 Serving
Total Time: 10 Minutes
Prep Time: 5 Minutes
Cook Time: 5 Minutes

Ingredients

- 50g oatmeal
- 15g chia seeds
- 40g chocolate protein powder
- 15g cacao powder
- 50ml almond milk
- 100ml water
- Natural peanut butter

Directions

In a pan, combine oatmeal and chai seeds; stir in water and cook on low heat for about 5 minutes, stirring frequently so that chia seeds don't stick together. Stir in chocolate protein powder and then stir in the remaining ingredients until well combined. Serve topped with smooth peanut butter.

Nutritional Information per Serving:
Calories: 466; Total Fat: 24.7 g; Carbs: 33.4 g; Dietary Fiber: 4.3 g; Sugars: 11.6g; Protein: 27.3 g; Cholesterol: 4 mg; Sodium: 299 mg

23. Mushroom & Tomato Omelet

Yield: 1 Serving

Total Time: 15 Minutes

Prep Time: 5 Minutes

Cook Time: 5 Minutes

Ingredients
- 2 eggs
- 10g butter
- 50g grated cheddar cheese
- 50g button mushrooms, chopped
- 2 tomatoes, chopped
- Pinch salt
- Pinch pepper

Directions

In a bowl, whisk together eggs, salt and pepper until well combined.

Melt butter in a skillet over medium heat and sauté red onion and mushroom until tender; pour in the egg mixture.

Cook, tilting the pan to allow the uncooked egg to flow on the empty sides of the pan. Sprinkle grated cheese over one half of the omelet and top with chopped tomatoes; with a spatula, fold the other half of the omelet over onto the filled half. Cook for a few seconds or until the cheese is melted and egg is set. Enjoy!

Nutritional Information per Serving:
Calories: 454; Total Fat: 34.1 g; Carbs: 12.7 g; Dietary Fiber: 3.5 g; Sugars: 8.3 g; Protein: 27.4 g; Cholesterol: 401 mg; Sodium: 661 mg

24. Healthy Coconut Pancakes

Yield: 1 Serving

Total Time: 20 Minutes

Prep Time: 10 Minutes

Cook Time: 10 Minutes

Ingredients

- 5g melted coconut oil
- 60ml coconut milk
- 50g coconut flour
- 1 egg
- 40g vanilla protein powder
- 1 tsp baking powder
- 1 pinch salt
- 5g coconut oil
- Blueberries

Directions

Separate the egg white from yolk and then using a hand mixer, whip the egg white together with salt until stiff peaks form; set aside.

In another bowl, whisk together coconut milk, oil and yolks until well combined; whisk in protein powder, baking powder and coconut flour until smooth. Fold egg whites in the batter and let stand for at least 5 minutes.

Melt coconut oil in a nonstick pan and then add batter; spread and cook the pancakes for about 2 minutes per side. Repeat until all the batter is used up.
Serve the pancakes with fresh berries. Enjoy!

Nutritional Information Per Serving Size
Calories: 460; Total Fat: 33.4 g; Carbs: 16.63 g; Dietary Fiber: 2.8g; Sugars: 5.1g; Protein: 27.8g; Cholesterol: 168mg; Sodium: 384mg;

25. Healthy Breakfast Casserole

Yield: 6 Servings

Total Time: 50 Minutes

Prep Time: 5 Minutes

Cook Time: 45 Minutes

Ingredients

- 1 tablespoon coconut oil
- 1/2 pound ground beef
- 1 large sweet potato, cut into slices
- 1/2 cup spinach
- 12 eggs
- Salt and pepper

Directions

Preheat oven to 350°F. Lightly coat a square baking tray with coconut oil and set aside.

In a skillet set over medium heat, brown ground beef in coconut oil; season well and remove from heat.
Layer the potato slices onto the baking tray and top with raw spinach and ground beef.
In a small bowl, whisk eggs, salt and pepper until well blended; pour over the mixture to cover completely; bake for about 45 minutes or until eggs are cooked

through and the potatoes are tender. Remove from oven and let cool a bit before serving.

Nutrition info Per Serving:
Calories: 247; Total Fat: 15.2 g; Carbs: 7 g; Dietary Fiber: 1.1 g; Sugars: 2.6; Protein: 22.1 g; Cholesterol: 366 mg; Sodium: 176 mg

26. Ginger Detox Smoothie

Yield: 1 Serving

Total Time: 5 Minutes

Prep Time: 5 Minutes

Cook Time: N/A

Ingredients:

- 1 cup Greek yogurt
- 1 inch fresh turmeric
- 1 cup spinach
- 1 inch fresh ginger
- 1 teaspoon cinnamon

Directions

Combine all ingredients in a blender and blend until very smooth. Enjoy!

27. Spicy Breakfast Carrot Pudding

Yield: 4 Servings

Total Time: 20 Minutes

Prep Time: 10 Minutes

Cook Time: 10 Minutes

Ingredients

- 1 cup light coconut milk
- 1 1/2 cups unsweetened almond milk
- 1 cup shredded carrots
- 1/4 teaspoon ground cloves
- 1/2 teaspoon ground cinnamon
- 1/4 teaspoon ground ginger
- 1/3 teaspoon ground cardamom
- 1 teaspoon vanilla extract
- 1 teaspoon liquid stevia
- 1/2 chia seeds

Directions

In a saucepan set over medium heat, combine ½ cup coconut milk, ½ cup almond milk and shredded carrots; stir in spices and cook for about 20 minutes or until carrots are tender. Remove from heat and set aside to cool.

Transfer the carrots along with cooking liquid to a blender and blend until very smooth.

Add stevia and the remaining milks and continue blending until combined; transfer to a large bowl and stir in chia seeds until well combined. Refrigerate for about 15 minutes, stirring, or until set. Serve into serving bowls topped with pumpkin seeds and toasted chopped walnuts.

Nutritional Information per Serving:

Calories: 419; Total Fat: 22.1 g; Crabs: 56.2 g; Dietary Fiber: 5.1 g; Sugars: 46.5 g; Protein: 3g; Cholesterol: 0 mg; Sodium: 92 mg

CHRON'S DIET LUNCH RECIPES

28.   Spinach & Turkey Soup

Yield: 1 Serving

Total Time: 10 Minutes

Prep Time: 10 Minutes

Cook Time: N/A

Ingredients

- 1 teaspoon extra-virgin olive oil
- 100 grams turkey, diced
- 1 clove garlic, minced
- 1 tablespoon chopped red onion
- ½ lemon with rind
- 1 stalk lemongrass
- ¼ teaspoon thyme
- Pinch of salt & pepper
- 2 cups chicken broth
- ¼ cup fresh lemon juice
- 2 cups chopped spinach

Directions

In a small saucepan brown the diced turkey in olive oil; stir in garlic, onion, herbs, spices, broth, lemon juice and lemon rind and simmer for about 20-30 minutes, adding spinach during the last 5 minutes. Serve hot.

Nutritional Information per Serving:
Calories: 240; Total Fat: 6 g; Carbs: 4.2 g; Dietary Fiber: 1.1 g; Sugars: 2 g; Protein: 39.7 g; Cholesterol: 77 mg; Sodium: 1614 mg

29. Healthy Beef Lettuce Wraps

Yields: 4 Servings

Total Time: 35 Minutes

Prep Time: 15 Minutes

Cook Time: 20 Minutes

Ingredients

- 1/2 lb. ground beef
- 1/2 small onion, finely chopped
- 1 garlic clove, minced
- 2 tablespoons extra virgin olive oil
- 1 head lettuce
- 1 teaspoon cumin
- 1/2 tablespoon fresh ginger, sliced
- 2 tablespoons freshly squeezed lime juice
- 2 tablespoons freshly chopped cilantro
- 1 teaspoon freshly ground black pepper
- 1 teaspoon sea salt

Directions

Sauté garlic and onion in extra virgin olive oil until fragrant and translucent.

Add ground beef and cook well.

Stir in the remaining ingredients and continue cooking for 5 minutes more.

To serve, ladle a spoonful of turkey mixture onto a lettuce leaf and wrap. Enjoy!

Nutrition Information per Serving:

Calories: 192; Total Fat: 13.6 g; Carbs: 4.6 g; Dietary Fiber: 1 g; Sugars: 1.2 g Protein: 16.3 g; Cholesterol: 58 mg; Sodium: 535 mg

30. Healthy Savory Beef Stew

Yield: 2 Servings
Total Time: 45 Minutes
Prep Time: 10 Minutes
Cook Time: 35 Minutes

Ingredients

- 1/2 lb. lean steak
- 1 clove garlic, minced
- 1 tablespoon chopped red onion
- 4 stalks celery, chopped
- 1 cup beef broth
- Pinch of oregano
- 1/8 teaspoon garlic powder
- 1/8 teaspoon onion powder
- Pinch of salt & pepper

Directions:
Brown beef, garlic and onion; stir in spices, veggies and water; bring to a boil and lower heat. Simmer for about 30 minutes or until beef is cooked through. Serve hot garnished with parsley.

Nutritional Information per Serving:
Calories: 217; Total Fat: 7 g; Saturated Fat: 2.6g; Carbs: 2.8 g; Dietary Fiber: 1.1 g; Sugars: 1.1 g; Protein: 35.7 g; Cholesterol: 89 mg; Sodium: 462 mg

31. Shrimp & Pineapple Curry

Yield: 4 Servings

Total Time: 25 Minutes

Prep Time: 10 Minutes

Cook Time: 15 Minutes

Ingredients
- 2 tablespoons coconut oil
- 60g yellow curry paste
- 400g diced pineapple
- 700g large shrimp peeled and deveined
- 250g coconut milk
- 1 banana
- 40g fish sauce
- 1 zucchini, diced
- 60g Thai basil and cilantro chopped
- 1 lime quartered

Directions

In a blender or food processor, blend together banana, fish sauce, and coconut milk until very smooth; set aside.

Heat oil in a skillet over medium heat and stir in yellow curry paste; cook for about 2 minutes. Add in pineapple and cook for about 3 minutes or until caramelized. Stir in shrimp and cook for about 2 minutes or until shrimp turns pink; transfer shrimp to a bowl and set aside. Add the coconut-banana mixture to the skillet and cook for about 3 minutes; stir in zucchini and cook for 2 minutes or until the sauce is thick. Return shrimp back to the skillet and stir in herbs. Cook until heated through and serve with sliced lime and more herbs. Enjoy!

Nutritional Information Per Serving:
Calories: 460; Total Fat: 25.9 g; Carbs: 34.8 g; Dietary Fiber: 11.6 g; sugars: 16.6 g; Protein: 29.1 g; Cholesterol: 221 mg; Sodium: 2069 mg

32. Lean Steak & Veggie in Coconut Curry Sauce

Yield: 4 Servings

Total Time: 30 Minutes

Prep Time: 10 Minutes

Cook Time: 20 Minutes

Ingredients:

- 250g lean steak
- 200g carrots, sliced
- 400g broccoli, cut into florets
- 400g fresh peas
- 3 garlic cloves, thinly sliced
- 2 medium onions, thinly sliced
- 250g vegetable stock
- 250g coconut milk
- 1 tablespoon coconut oil
- 1 tablespoon fresh lemon juice
- 10g grated lemon peel
- 20g curry powder
- Freshly ground black pepper

Directions

Heat oil in a pan; sauté garlic, onion and curry powder for about 3 minutes. Stir in beef and cook for about 5 minutes per side or until browned. Add carrots, broccoli, peas, and salt; fry for a few minutes and then stir in stock, coconut milk, and lemon peel; cover and cook for about 30 minutes or until the veggies are tender and beef is cooked through.
Serve.

Nutritional Information per Serving:
Calories: 419; Total Fat: 22.5g; Carbs: 30.8g; Dietary Fiber: 13.4g; Sugars: 11.6g; Protein: 29.9g; Cholesterol: 48mg; Sodium: 579mg

33. Healthy Protein-Packed Fish Tikka Curry

Yield: 4 Servings

Total Time: 1 Hour 30 Minutes

Prep Time: 10 Minutes

Cook Time: 1 Hour 20 Minutes

Ingredients

- Juice of half lemon
- Wedges of half lemon
- 3 tablespoons tikka curry paste
- 400g cod fish fillets
- 1 onion, sliced
- 2 cloves of garlic, sliced
- 1 thumb-sized piece of ginger, sliced
- 1 fresh red chili, chopped
- 15 g fresh coriander, chopped
- 1 tablespoon olive oil
- 200g potatoes, diced into 2cm chunks
- 200g ripe tomatoes, diced
- 200g frozen cauliflower florets
- 50g red split lentils
- 150 g basmati rice
- 10 cloves
- 100g fat-free natural yoghurt

Directions

On a large plate, mix 1 tablespoon of tikka paste and lemon juice until well combined; massage the mixture over the fish and set aside to marinate.

In a casserole pan set over medium heat, mix garlic, onion, ginger, coriander, chili, oil and the remaining tikka paste; stir in the potatoes and cook for about 15 minutes or until tender.

Stir in cauliflower, tomatoes, lentil and 600ml boiling water; bring to a gentle boil. Simmer for about 45 minutes until lentils are tender and the sauce is thick. Season.

Meanwhile, in a pan, combine 1 cup rice and 2 cups boiling water; stir in cloves and salt and cook over medium heat for about 12 minutes or until water is absorbed and rice is tender.

In a large nonstick pan, dry fry fish for about 5 minutes per side or until cooked through and charred on the outside.

Stir yogurt into the curry and fluff rice. Serve rice on a platter and flake fish on top; garnish with coriander and lemon wedges. Serve alongside the curry.

Nutritional Information Per Serving:
Calories: 391; Total Fat: 6.9 g; Carbs: 55.8 g; Dietary Fiber: 8 g; sugars: 4.8 g; Protein: 29.2 g; Cholesterol: 54 mg; Sodium: 395 mg

34. Protein Chicken Curry with Coconut Rice

Yield: 2 Servings

Total Time: 40 Minutes

Prep Time: 10 Minutes

Cook Time: 30 Minutes

Ingredients

- 200g skinless boneless chicken thighs, diced
- 1 small onion, sliced
- 100g eggplant, diced
- 1 tsp grated ginger
- 1 sliced green chilli
- 1 garlic clove, sliced
- 1 teaspoon curry powder
- 1 teaspoon graham. masala
- 100g chopped plum tomatoes
- 100g water
- 100 coconut milk
- 100g white rice
- 2 cardamom pods, bashed

Directions

Heat oil in a skillet and sauté eggplant and chicken for about 5 minutes or until chicken is lightly browned; stir in onion, garlic, ginger, chili, spices and tomatoes. Add a splash of water and simmer, covered, for about 15 minutes or until chicken is cooked through and the sauce is thickened

In another pan, combine water, coconut milk, rice and cardamom pods; bring to a gentle boil and then simmer for about 10 minutes or until rice is tender and the liquid is absorbed. Serve the rice topped with the chicken curry. Enjoy!

Nutritional Information per Serving:
Calories: 468; Total Fat: 16.5g; Carbs: 52.2g; Dietary Fiber: 6.5g; Sugars: 7.2g; Protein: 29.5g; Cholesterol: 73mg; Sodium: 68mg

35. Gut Healing Soup

Yield: 4 Servings

Total Time: 40 Minutes

Prep Time: 15 Minutes

Cook Time: 25 Minutes

Ingredients

- 1 tablespoon coconut oil
- 1 cup chopped red onion
- 2 cloves of garlic, minced
- 2 stalks celery, chopped
- 2 parsnips, sliced
- 3 carrots, sliced
- 4 cups diced shitake mushrooms
- 4 cups homemade vegetable broth
- 11/2 teaspoons freshly grated ginger
- 2 small bay leaves
- 1 teaspoon black peppercorns
- 1/2 teaspoon ground turmeric
- 2 cups fresh lemon juice
- Handful chopped fresh parsley

Directions

In a large stockpot, combine homemade vegetable broth, ginger, bay leaves, peppercorns, and turmeric; bring the mixture to a rolling boil; cover and simmer for about 3 minutes; strain the soup to remove peppercorns and bay leaves.

In a skillet, melt coconut oil and sauté in red onions, garlic, celery, parsnips, and carrots for about 5 minutes or until fragrant; stir in sea salt and pepper and then remove from heat. Stir in stir in shiitake mushrooms and the broth mixture. Cook for about 5 minutes or until the mushrooms are crisp tender. Remove from heat and stir in fresh lemon juice.

Serve warm.

36. Delicious Low Carb Chicken Curry

Yield: 1 Serving

Total Time: 30 Minutes

Prep Time: 10 Minutes

Cook Time: 20 Minutes

Ingredients
- 100 grams chicken, diced
- ¼ cup chicken broth
- Pinch of turmeric
- Dash of onion powder
- 1 tablespoon minced red onion
- Pinch of garlic powder
- ¼ teaspoon curry powder
- Pinch of sea salt
- Pinch of pepper
- Stevia, optional
- Pinch of cayenne

Directions

In a small saucepan, stir spices in chicken broth until dissolved; stir in chicken, garlic, onion, and stevia and cook until chicken is cooked through and liquid is reduced by half. Serve hot.

Nutritional Information per Serving:
Calories: 170; Total Fat: 3.5 g; Carbs: 2.3 g; Dietary Fiber: 0.6 g; Sugars: 0.8 g; Protein: 30.5 g; Cholesterol: 77 mg; Sodium: 255 mg

37. Zucchini & Mushroom Soup

Yield: 8 Servings

Total Time: 35 Minutes

Prep Time: 10 Minutes

Cook Time: 25 Minutes

Ingredients

- 1 tablespoon extra-virgin olive oil
- 1/2 small onion, chopped
- 1/4 teaspoon ground turmeric
- 3 cloves garlic, minced
- 1 teaspoon minced ginger
- 1 cup chopped celery
- 1 cup sliced shiitake mushrooms
- 1 cup chopped large carrots
- 1 cup chopped zucchini
- 1 1/2 chopped cauliflower
- 4 cups vegetable broth
- 4 tablespoons fresh lemon juice
- 1/2 teaspoon cayenne pepper
- 1/2 teaspoon black pepper
- 1/2 teaspoon sea salt
- 1 cup Greek yogurt, to serve

Directions

Heat olive oil in a large pot set over medium heat; sauté red onion, garlic, turmeric, and ginger for about 4 minutes. Stir in the remaining veggies, salt and pepper and cook for 5 minutes; stir in fresh lemon juice, broth, and cayenne pepper and cook for about 15 minutes or until the veggies are tender.Transfer the mixture to a food processor and process until very smooth and creamy. Serve the soup topped with a dollop of Greek yogurt. Enjoy!

Nutritional Information per Servings:

Calories: 57; Total Fat: 11 g; Carbs: 9 g; Dietary Fiber: 1 g; Sugars: 3 g; Protein: 1 g; Cholesterol: 70 mg; Sodium: 498 mg

38. Lettuce Avocado & Egg Salad Wraps

Yield: 4 Servings

Prep Time: 10 minutes

Total Time: 10 minutes

Cook Time: N/A

Ingredients

- 4 eggs boiled, sliced
- 1 medium avocado, diced
- 2 teaspoons lemon juice
- 3 tablespoons mayonnaise
- 2 tablespoons chives finely chopped
- 1/2 teaspoons salt
- 1/4 teaspoon pepper
- 8 leaves baby lettuce or romaine

Directions

In a bowl, combine sliced eggs and avocado.
In a small bowl, whisk together mayonnaise, lemon juice, chives, salt and pepper until well blended; pour over the avocado egg mixture and toss to coat well. Add a quarter cup of the avocado mixture onto each lettuce leaf and fold to wrap. Enjoy!

Nutritional Information per Serving:

Calories: 136; Total Fat: 12g; Carbs: 0.7g; Dietary Fiber: 0.6g; Sugars: 0g; Protein: 5g; Cholesterol: 168mg; Sodium: 419mg

39. Grilled Shiitake Mushrooms

Yield: 4 Servings

Total Time: 20 Minutes

Prep Time: 10 Minutes

Cook Time: 10 Minutes

Ingredients

- 2 cups shiitake mushrooms
- 1 tablespoon balsamic vinegar
- 1/4 cup extra virgin olive oil
- 1-2 garlic cloves, minced
- A handful of parsley
- 1 teaspoon salt

Directions

Rinse the mushroom and pat dry; put in a foil and drizzle with balsamic vinegar and extra virgin olive oil. Sprinkle the mushroom with garlic, parsley, and salt. Grill for about 10 minutes or until tender and cooked through. Serve warm.

Nutritional Information per Serving:

Calories: 171; Total Fat: 12.8g; Carbs: 15.9g; Dietary Fiber: 2.4g; Protein: 1.8g; Cholesterol: 0mg; Sodium: 854mg; sugars: 4.1g

40. Healthy Savory Beef Stew with Avocado

Yield: 2 Servings

Total Time: 45 Minutes

Prep Time: 10 Minutes

Cook Time: 35 Minutes

Ingredients
- 150 lean steak
- 1 clove garlic, minced
- 20g chopped red onion
- 4 stalks celery, chopped
- 250g beef or chicken broth
- Pinch of cayenne
- Pinch of oregano
- 1/8 teaspoon garlic powder
- 1/8 teaspoon onion powder
- Pinch of salt & pepper
- 1 avocado, diced

Directions:

Brown beef, garlic and onion; stir in spices, veggies and coconut milk; bring to a boil and lower heat. Simmer for about 30 minutes or until beef is cooked through. Serve hot topped with avocado and garnished with parsley.

Nutritional Information per Serving:

Calories: 395; Total Fat: 18.1g; Saturated Fat:34.2g; Carbs: 2.8 g; Dietary Fiber: 9.1 g; Sugars: 3 g; Protein: 28.2 g; Cholesterol: 60 mg; Sodium: 798 mg

41. Italian Fish Stew with Yummy Mashed Potatoes

Yield: 4 Servings

Total Time: 55 Minutes

Prep Time: 10 Minutes

Cook Time: 45 Minutes

Ingredients

- 550g Kingklip fish fillets
- 2 onions, finely chopped
- 4 garlic cloves, minced
- 100g peeled, chopped tomato
- 40g tomato paste
- 250g white wine
- ½ tsp. parsley, chopped
- ¼ tsp. dried oregano
- salt and pepper to taste
- 4 tablespoons olive oil
- 2 cups water
- 400g potatoes, diced

Directions

Preheat oven to 360C

Sauté onion and garlic on a pot then add tinned tomatoes and tomato paste and stir.

Pour the wine, parsley, oregano, salt, pepper, and water. Stir well and bring to a simmer. Let it simmer for 10-15 minutes to reduce and thicken. Meanwhile, place your fish in baking dish. When sauce is nice and thick, pour it over fish and sprinkle with a little extra oregano. Cover the dish with foil and place in the oven to cook for 20 minutes. Take foil off and return to oven uncovered and cook for another 10 minutes. Boil potatoes in a pot of salted boiling water until tender; mash until smooth. Serve the fish stew over the mash. Enjoy!

Nutritional Information per Serving:
Calories: 394; Total Fat: 14.9g; Saturated Fat:37g; Carbs: 2.8g; Dietary Fiber: 5.1g; Sugars: 13.2g; Protein: 29.5g; Cholesterol: 59 mg; Sodium: 111 mg

42. Lean Steak & Mung Cleansing Soup

Yield: 3 Servings

Total Time: 20 Minutes

Prep Time: 5 Minutes

Cook Time: 15 Minutes

Ingredients

- 300g lean steak
- 2 teaspoon sesame oil
- 50g diced carrots
- 50g chopped celery
- 100g chopped leeks or onions
- 2 garlic cloves, minced
- 1 teaspoon minced ginger
- 1 tablespoon date paste
- 30g nut paste (walnuts and pumpkin seeds)
- 2 teaspoons lemon/lime juice
- 1 teaspoon allspice
- 1/4 teaspoon cardamom powder
- 2 teaspoons cumin powder
- A pinch of red chili flakes
- 1/2 teaspoon crushed black pepper
- Salt
- 1 kg vegetable broth
- 200g coarsely chopped spinach
- 200g cooked yellow mung beans
- 1 ½ avocado, diced

Directions

Heat oil in a stock pot over medium high heat; fry beef until browned on both sides. Stir in chopped veggies and seasonings except spinach. Cook for about 10 minutes and then stir in, vegetable broth, spinach and mung beans; simmer for about 3 minutes and remove from heat.

Transfer the mixture to a food processor and blend until the soup is smooth. Serve the soup with small avocado cubes, garnished with tomatoes and parsley.

Nutritional Information per Serving:
Calories: 437; Total Fat: 38.7 g; Carbs: 39.6 g; Dietary Fiber: 8.9 g; Sugars: 5.2 g; Protein: 29.1 g; Cholesterol: 60 mg; Sodium: 153 mg

43. Sauteed Green Bean & Zucchini Bowl

Yield: 2 Servings

Total Time: 15 Minutes

Prep Time: 5 Minutes

Cook Time: 10 Minutes

Ingredients

- 2 tablespoons extra virgin olive oil, divided
- 1/4 cup green beans - cut into small pieces
- ½ small zucchini, thinly sliced
- A pinch of salt
- 2 tablespoons lemon juice
- 2 tablespoons sliced scallions

Directions

Add half of the oil to a skillet set over medium heat. Stir in green beans, zucchini, and salt and sauté, stirring, for about 9 minutes or until the veggies are crisp tender.

Remove the pan from heat and stir in lemon juice and scallions. Serve immediately.

Nutritional Information per Serving:

Calories: 46; Total Fat: 3.7g; Carbs: 3.4g; Dietary Fiber: 1.4g; Protein: 1g; Cholesterol: 0mg; Sodium: 200mg; sugars: 1.1g

44. Lemony Squash Salad

Yield: 4 Servings

Total Time: 10 Minutes

Prep Time: 10 Minutes

Cook Time: N/A

Ingredients

- 1/2 cup thinly sliced red onion
- 2 scallions, sliced
- 1 cup steamed baby spinach
- 2 cups cooked teff
- 1 medium yellow squash, diced
- 1 teaspoon balsamic vinegar
- 3 tablespoons fresh lemon juice
- 1 tablespoon lemon zest
- 1/2 teaspoon sea salt
- 1/4 teaspoon freshly ground black pepper
- 2 teaspoons ground chia seeds
- 1 large head Bibb lettuce, coarsely chopped into pieces
- 1 tablespoon chopped cilantro

Directions

Mix red onion, scallions, spinach, teff and squash in a large bowl. In a small bowl, whisk together vinegar, lemon juice, lemon zest, sea salt, pepper and chia seeds until well combined; pour over the teff mixture and toss to coat well. Place lettuce pieces into serving bowls and evenly divide the teff mixture on top; serve garnished with cilantro.

Nutritional Information per Serving:
Calories: 248 Total Fat: 2.2 g; Carbs: 48.3 g; Dietary Fiber: 9.4 g; Sugars: 2 g; Protein: 9.2 g; Cholesterol: 0 mg; Sodium: 259 mg

45. Tasty Bean Soup with Tortilla Chips

Yield: 6 Servings

Total Time: 1 Hour 10 Minutes

Prep Time: 10 Minutes

Cook Time: 1 Hour

Ingredients

- 6 cups boiling water
- 1 large red onion, diced
- 1 pound dried black beans
- 1/4 teaspoon chipotle chile powder
- 2 teaspoons cumin
- 1 teaspoon sea salt
- 1 cup salsa
- 1 tablespoon fresh lime juice
- Avocado slices
- baked tortilla chips

Directions

Boil water in an instant pot and turn it to sauté setting; add onion and cook, stirring often, until tender and browned. Stir in beans, chipotle chili powder, cumin, boiling water, and sea salt; turn off the sauté function. Lock lid in place and turn on high pressure, adjusting time to 30 minutes. Let pressure come down naturally before opening the pot. Remove about 3 cups of beans to a blender and blend until very smooth; return to pot and add salsa. Adjust seasoning and turn the pot on sauté; cook until heated through. Ladle in serving bowls and drizzle with lime juice, garnish with avocado slices and serve with baked tortilla chips.

Nutritional Information per Serving:
Calories: 329; Total Fat: 1 g; Carbs: 65 g; Dietary Fiber: 9.3 g; Sugars: 7 g; Protein: 18 g; Cholesterol: 0 mg; Sodium: 707 mg

46. Vegan Red Lentil Soup

Yield: 6 Servings

Total Time: 45 Minutes

Prep Time: 10 Minutes

Cook Time: 35 Minutes

Ingredients

- 6 cups low-sodium vegetable broth
- 2 tablespoons minced garlic
- 1 1/2 cups chopped red onion
- 1 teaspoon paprika
- 1 teaspoon ground coriander
- ½ teaspoon ground pepper
- 1 1/2 cups red lentils
- 1 1/2-2 cups chopped carrots
- Fresh lemon juice
- Fresh cilantro, chopped

Directions

Add vegetable stock to a saucepan and stir in garlic, onion, paprika, coriander and ground pepper; bring to a gentle boil. Boil for about 5 minutes and then add in lentils; simmer for about 15 minutes and then add in chopped carrots.

Cook, covered, for 15 minutes more or until lentils are tender. Blend in a food processor until very smooth. Serve in bowls garnished with fresh lemon and chopped cilantro. Enjoy!

Nutrition Information per Serving
Calories: 213; Total Fat: 0.6 g; Carbs: 36.5 g; Dietary Fiber: 6.2 g; Sugars: 3.6 g; Protein: 15.2 g Cholesterol: 0 mg; Sodium: 94 mg

47. Lunch Salad with Lemony Dressing

Yield: 6 Servings

Total Time: 10 Minutes

Prep Time: 10 Minutes

Cook Time: N/A

Ingredients

For Lemony Poppy Seed Dressing

- ½ cup fresh lemon juice
- 6 tablespoons water
- ½-inch knob of ginger, minced
- 1 tablespoon Dijon mustard
- 1½ tablespoons maple syrup
- 1 clove garlic, chopped
- ¼ teaspoon salt
- ¼ teaspoon Pepper
- 1 tablespoon poppy seeds

For the Salad

- 1 cup carrots, roughly chopped
- 2 cups red cabbage, roughly chopped
- 2 cups Brussels sprouts, roughly chopped
- 2 cups broccoli florets
- 2 cups kale
- 2 tablespoons toasted sunflower seeds
- ½ cup almonds, chopped
- ½ cup chopped parsley

Directions

In a blender, blend together all the ingredients, except poppy seeds until smooth; add poppy seeds and set aside.

Mix all the salad ingredients in a large bowl; drizzle with the dressing and toss to coat well. Serve.

Nutrition Information per Serving

Calories: 175; Total Fat: 11.8 g; Carbs: 15.4 g; Dietary Fiber; 4.7 g; Sugars: 5.6 g; Protein: 5.3 g Cholesterol: 0 mg; Sodium: 27 mg

48. Chickpea Salad Wrap

Yield: 3 Servings

Total Time: 5 Minutes

Prep Time: 5 Minutes

Cook Time: N/A

Ingredients:

- 1 ½ cups cooked chickpeas
- 1/4 cup toasted sunflower seeds
- 1 tablespoon minced fresh dill
- 3 tablespoons chopped dill pickle
- 2 tablespoons chopped red onion
- 1/2 cup chopped celery
- 2 tablespoons fresh lemon juice
- 1/2 tsp regular mustard
- 1 garlic clove, minced
- ¼ teaspoon sea salt
- ¼ teaspoon pepper
- Wheat wraps

Directions:

In a large bowl, mix all the ingredients, mashing the chickpeas until smooth. Stuff the mixture into a wrap and serve.

Nutritional Information per Serving:

Calories: 302 Total Fat: 6.3 g; Carbs: 48.2 g; Dietary Fiber: 14 g; Sugars: 8.8 g; Protein: 15.6 g; Cholesterol: 0 mg; Sodium: 237 mg

49. Mango & Grilled Steak Salad w/ Buttermilk-Avocado Buttermilk Dressing

Yield: 4 Servings

Total Time: 10 Minutes

Prep Time: 10 Minutes

Cook Time: N/A

Ingredients

For the salads

- Salad greens
- 2 plum tomatoes, sliced
- 1 mango, thinly sliced
- Leftover steak, sliced thinly

Dressing

- 2/3 cup buttermilk
- half of an avocado
- 8-10 chives
- 1 clove of garlic, chopped
- 4 fresh basil leaves
- 1 teaspoon dried minced red onion
- A sprig fresh rosemary
- 1/2 teaspoon dried dill
- A few leaves of fresh parsley

- 1/2 liquid stevia
- pinch of chicory powder
- 1/4 teaspoon sea salt
- Pinch of pepper

Directions

Mix salad ingredients and divide among serving plates; top each with steak slices, tomato, and mango.

In a food processor or blend, blend together dressing ingredients until very smooth; pour over salad and toss to coat well. Enjoy!

Nutritional Information per Serving:
Calories: 34; Total Fat: 11.2 g; Carbs: 23 g; Dietary Fiber: 4.5 g; Sugars: 16.1 g; Protein: 38.8 g; Cholesterol: 1.3 mg; Sodium: 311 mg

Tasty Lime Cilantro Cauliflower Rice

Yield: 5 Servings

Total Time: 30 minutes

Prep Time: 20 Minutes

Cook Time: 10 Minutes

Ingredients:

- 1 head cauliflower, rinsed
- 1 tablespoon extra-virgin olive oil
- 2 garlic cloves, minced
- 2 scallions, chopped
- ½ teaspoon sea salt
- Pinch of pepper
- 4 tablespoons fresh lime juice
- 1/4 cup chopped fresh cilantro

Directions:

Chop cauliflower into florets and transfer to a food processor; pulse into rice texture.

Heat a large skillet over medium heat and add olive oil; sauté garlic and scallions for about 4 minutes or until fragrant and tender. Increase heat to medium high and stir in cauliflower rice; cook, covered, for about 6 minutes or until cauliflower is crispy on outside and soft inside. Season with salt and pepper and transfer to a bowl. Toss with freshly squeezed lime juice and cilantro and serve right away.

Nutrition Information per Serving:

Calories: 61; Total Fat: 3 g; Carbs: 8 g; Dietary Fiber: 3 g; Sugars: 0 g; Protein: 2.5 g; Cholesterol: 0 mg; Sodium: 37 mg

50. Turmeric Chickpea & Artichoke Sauté

Yield: 4 Servings

Total Time: 12 Minutes

Prep Time: 5 Minutes

Cook Time: 7 Minutes

Ingredients
- 3 tablespoons extra virgin olive oil
- 1 ½ cup artichoke hearts
- 1 ½ cup cooked chickpeas
- 1 tablespoon minced garlic
- 1 teaspoon coriander
- 2 teaspoons turmeric
- 1 teaspoon fenugreek seeds
- 1 teaspoon shaved ginger
- ½ teaspoon sea salt
- ½ teaspoon pepper

Directions

Heat a cast iron over medium high heat.

In a bowl, mix together olive oil, artichoke hearts, chickpeas and seasoning; toss into the hot skillet for about 6 minutes or until chickpeas are browned. Serve drizzled with fresh lemon juice.

Nutrition Information per Serving:
Calories: 224; Total Fat: 12 g; Carbs: 23 g; Dietary Fiber: 8 g; Sugars: 4 g Protein: 7 g; Cholesterol: 0 mg; Sodium: 541 mg

51. Crunchy Salmon Arugula Salad

Yield: 1 Serving

Total Time: 15 Minutes

Prep Tip Time: 5 Minutes

Cook Time: 10 Minutes

Ingredients

- 3 ounce wild-caught salmon fillet
- 2 small radishes, sliced thinly
- ¼ cup cucumber, diced
- 1 cup arugula leaves
- ¼ cup orange segments
- ¼ cup extra-virgin olive oil
- 1 tablespoon fresh lemon juice
- 1 tablespoon Dijon mustard
- 1 tsp herbes de provence spices
- Pinch of sea salt
- Pinch of pepper

Directions

Heat a tablespoon of olive oil in a skillet over medium high heat; sprinkle fish with salt and pepper and place in the pan, skin-side down. Cook for about 4 minutes per side or until cooked through and browned. Meanwhile, combine sliced radish, cucumber, arugula, and orange segments in a salad bowl. In a small bowl, whisk together fresh lemon juice, mustard, herbes de provence and remaining olive oil until well blended.

Place fish over the salad and drizzle with the dressing. Serve right away.

Nutrition Information per Serving:

Calories: 556; Total Fat: 39 g; Carbs: 35 g; Dietary Fiber: 1 g; Sugars: 9 g Protein: 19 g; Cholesterol: 45 mg; Sodium: 644 mg

52. Delicious African Beef Curry

Yield: 6 Servings

Total Time: 2 Hours 30 Minutes

Prep Time: 10 Minutes

Cook Time: 2 Hours 20 Minutes

Ingredients
- 600g boned lean beef chuck
- 2 onions, chopped
- 300g Roma tomatoes, chopped
- 500g beef broth
- 1 teaspoon turmeric
- 15g minced garlic
- 10g mustard seed
- 10g curry powder
- 10g minced jalapeño chilies
- 10g minced ginger
- 300g hot cooked rice
- 100g mango chutney
- 1 banana, thinly sliced
- 60g yogurt
- 30g shredded dried coconut
- 1 teaspoon salt

Directions

In a skillet, combine onions, beef and a cup of water; cover and bring a gentle boil and then simmer for about 30 minutes. Uncover and cook on high for about 7 minutes or until all the liquid evaporates and onions and beef are browned. Stir in garlic, mustard seeds, curry powder and turmeric and cook for about 1 minute or until spices are fragrant. Stir in ginger, chilies, tomatoes, and broth and simmer for about 2 hours. Ladle the curry over rice and top each serving with banana, coconut, chutney, and yogurt. Sprinkle each with salt and enjoy!

Nutritional Information per Serving:

Calories: 434; Total Fat: 10.4g; Carbs: 58.72g; Dietary Fiber: 5.8g; Sugars: 11g; Protein: 28.6g; Cholesterol: 76mg; Sodium: 863mg

CHRON'S DIET DINNER RECIPES

53. Sweet Potato & Herbed Chicken Casserole

Yield: 4 Servings

Total Time: 60 Minutes

Prep Time: 15 Minutes

Cook Time: 45 Minutes

Ingredients

- 4 tablespoons herbs mix: basil, oregano, thyme and rosemary, thyme, oregano, basil
- 2 tablespoons garlic powder
- 1/2 cup extra-virgin olive oil
- Pinch of sea salt
- Pinch of pepper
- 2 pounds boneless chicken, diced
- 2 heads of broccoli, chopped
- 4 sweet potatoes, diced

Directions

Preheat oven to 400°F.

Whisk together herb mixture, garlic powder, olive oil, sea salt and pepper; stir in chicken, broccoli, and sweet potatoes until well coated; transfer the mixture to a casserole dish and bake for about 45 minutes, stirring after every 10 minutes.

Nutrition Information per Serving:

Calories: 736; Total Fat: 36 g; Carbs: 50 g; Dietary Fiber: 12 g; Sugars: 12 g Protein: 59 g; Cholesterol: 184 mg; Sodium: 368 mg

54. Chili Fried Steak with Toasted Cashews

Yields: 4 Servings

Total Time: 35 Minutes

Prep Time: 10 Minutes

Cook Time: 25 Minutes

Ingredients

- ½ tbsp. extra virgin olive oil or canola oil
- 1 pound sliced lean beef
- 2 tablespoons freshly squeezed lime juice
- 2 teaspoon fish sauce
- 2 teaspoons red curry paste
- 1 cup green capsicum, diced
- 24 toasted cashews
- 1 teaspoon arrowroot
- 1 teaspoon liquid stevia
- ½ cup water

Directions

Add oil to a pan set over medium heat; add beef and fry until it is no longer pink inside. Stir in red curry paste and cook for a few more minutes. Stir in stevia, lime juice, fish sauce, capsicum and water; simmer for about 10 minutes.

Mix cooked arrowroot with water to make a paste; stir the paste into the sauce to thicken it.

Remove the pan from heat and add toasted cashews. Serve.

Nutrition Information per Serving:
Calories: 252; Total Fat: 9.7 g; Carbs: 4 g; Dietary Fiber: 0.6 g; Sugars: 2.1 g Protein: 35.1 g; Cholesterol: 101 mg; Sodium: 441 mg

55. Grilled Chicken with Fresh Herb Marinade

Yield: 4 Servings

Total Time: 40 Minutes

Prep Time: 10 Minutes

Cook Time: 30 Minutes

Ingredients

- 1 cup chopped mixed fresh herb leaves (basil, parsley, cilantro)
- 2 large garlic cloves, chopped
- 1/4 cup lemon juice
- 1/4 cup extra-virgin olive oil
- 3 teaspoons sea salt
- 1/4 teaspoon pepper
- 1 pound chicken breasts, boneless, skinless, sliced in half lengthwise

Directions

In a food processor, process together herbs, garlic, lemon juice, oil, salt and pepper until smooth; transfer to a Ziploc bag and add chicken.

Shake to coat chicken well and refrigerate for about 30 minutes; grill the chicken for about 15 minutes per side or until cooked through.

Nutrition Information per Serving:

Calories: 183; Total Fat: 8 g; Carbs: 0 g; Dietary Fiber: 0 g; Sugars: 0 g Protein: 26 g; Cholesterol: 65 mg; Sodium: 73 mg

56. Salmon Served with Mashed Potatoes

Yields: 2 Servings

Total Time: 30 Minutes

Prep Time: 10 Minutes

Cook Time: 20 Minutes

Ingredients

- ¼ teaspoon thyme
- ¼ teaspoon basil
- ¼ teaspoon oregano
- ¼ teaspoon onion powder
- 2 teaspoons salt
- ¼ teaspoon white pepper
- ¼ teaspoon ground cayenne pepper
- ¼ teaspoon ground paprika
- 5 ounces tilapia fillet, skin and bones removed
- 2 teaspoons extra virgin olive oil
- 2 servings of mashed potatoes

Directions

Combine oregano, basil, thyme, white pepper, salt, onion powder, cayenne pepper, and paprika in a small bowl.

Brush fish with half of oil and sprinkle with the spice mixture. Drizzle with the remaining oil and cook fish in a skillet set over high heat until blackened and flakes easily with a fork. Serve with mashed potatoes.

Nutritional Information per Serving:

Calories: 188; Total Fat: 6.1 g; Carbs: 19 g; Dietary Fiber: 1.2g; Protein: 15.1 g; Cholesterol: 35 mg; Sodium: 2352 mg; sugars: trace

57. Grilled Steak Salad with Red Onion, Orange & Avocado

Yield: 4 Servings

Total Time: 15 Minutes

Prep Time: 15 Minutes

Cook Time: N/A

Ingredients

- 350g steak
- 2 tablespoons of canola oil
- Salt and pepper
- 2 tablespoons extra-virgin olive oil
- 1 small clove garlic, finely chopped
- 2 tablespoons sherry vinegar
- 2 medium navel oranges, segmented and segments squeezed into juice
- 1 teaspoon Dijon mustard
- 1/8 teaspoon salt
- 2 medium avocados, sliced
- 1/2 medium red onion, thinly sliced
- 300g Romaine lettuce, chopped

Directions

Brush the steak with canola oil and sprinkle with salt and pepper; grill on high for about 8 minutes per side or until cooked through and golden browned on both sides. Remove from heat and let rest for about 5 minutes before slicing to serve.
In a bowl, combine oil, garlic, vinegar, 1 tablespoon of orange juice, mustard and salt; whisk in extra virgin olive oil until smooth and emulsified.
In a salad bowl, combine sliced steak, avocado, red onion, lettuce, and strained orange segments; drizzle with the dressing and toss until well combined. Serve right away.

Nutritional Information per Serving:

Calories: 475; Total Fat: 33.2g; Carbs: 20.1g; Dietary Fiber: 9.2g; Sugars: 7.1g; Protein: 29.2g; Cholesterol: 57mg; Sodium: 481mg; sugars: 7g

58. Super Tasty Mushroom Marinara with Pasta

Yield: 2 Servings

Total Time: 45 Minutes

Prep Time: 10 Minutes

Cook Time: 35 Minutes

Ingredients:

- 1/2 cup water
- ½ cup chopped red onion
- 3-4 cups sliced mushrooms
- 2 garlic cloves, minced
- 1/2 teaspoon fennel seeds
- 1/8 teaspoon cayenne pepper
- 1 teaspoon dried thyme
- 1 teaspoon dried oregano
- 1 teaspoon dried basil
- 4 cups tomato sauce
- 2 cups chopped tomatoes
- 1 pound pasta

Directions:

Cook red onions in water for about 2 minutes; stir in mushrooms and garlic and cook for about 5 minutes or until mushrooms are lightly browned and onion is tender.

Stir in fennels seeds, cayenne, thyme, oregano, basil, tomato sauce and tomato and simmer for about 30 minutes.

Follow package instructions to cook pasta until tender; drain and serve topped with the mushroom sauce. Enjoy!

Nutrition Information per Serving
Calories: 194; Total Fat: 1.8 g; Carbs: 41.6 g; Dietary Fiber: 7.2 g; Sugars: 28.7 g; Protein: 12.1 g Cholesterol: 0 mg; Sodium: 2587 mg

59. Stir Fried Beef with Veggies

Yield: 4 Servings

Total Time: 20 Minutes

Prep Time: 10 Minutes

Cook Time: 10 Minutes

Ingredients:

- 1 pound grass-fed flank steak, thinly sliced strips
- 1 tablespoon rice wine
- 2 teaspoons balsamic vinegar
- Pinch of sea salt
- pinch of pepper
- 3 teaspoons extra-virgin olive oil
- 1 large yellow onion, thinly chopped
- 1/2 red bell pepper, thinly sliced
- 1/2 green bell pepper, thinly sliced
- 1 tablespoon toasted sesame seeds
- 1 teaspoon crushed red pepper flakes

Directions:

Place meat in a bowl; stir in rice wine and vinegar, sea salt and pepper. Toss to coat well.

Heat a tablespoon of olive oil in a pan set over medium high heat; add meat and cook for about 1 minute or until meat is browned; stir for another 2 minutes and then remove from heat. Heat the remaining oil to the pan and sauté onions for about 2 minutes or until caramelized; stir in pepper and cook for 2 minutes more; return meat to pan and stir in sesame seeds and red pepper flakes. Serve hot!

Nutritional Information per Serving:
Calories: 296; Total Fat: 14.3 g; Carbs: 8.3 g; Dietary Fiber: 1.6 g; Sugars: 4.2 g; Protein: 32.76 g; Cholesterol: 62 mg; Sodium: 157 mg

60. Creamy Citrus Salmon Baked in Coconut Milk

Yields: 4 Servings

Total Time: 35 Minutes

Prep Time: 15 Minutes

Cook Time: 25 Minutes

Ingredients

- 1 teaspoon coconut oil
- 4 salmon fillets
- 3 tablespoons freshly squeezed lemon juice
- 3 tablespoons freshly squeezed lime juice
- 3 tablespoons freshly squeezed orange juice
- 1 cup coconut milk
- 1 teaspoon ground pepper
- 1 teaspoon sea salt
- 1 teaspoon dried parsley flakes
- 1 finely chopped clove garlic

Directions

Preheat your oven to 190°C (275°F). Coat a baking dish with coconut oil.

Rinse the fish under water and pat dry with paper towels. Melt coconut oil in a skillet set over medium heat and add in salmon fish; cook for about 5 minutes per side of until browned on both sides. Transfer the fish fillet to the coated baking dish and drizzle with coconut milk, lemon, lime, and orange juices. Sprinkle with ground pepper, sea salt, parsley, and garlic. Bake in the oven for about 15 minutes or until the flakes easily when touched with a fork. Serve with a bowl of cooked brown rice or quinoa.

Nutritional Information per Serving:
Calories: 248; Total Fat: 12g; Carbs: 0.7g; Dietary Fiber: trace; Protein: 34.8g; Cholesterol: 0mg; Sodium: 82mg; trace

61. Tilapia with Mushroom Sauce

Yields: 4 Servings

Total Time: 35 Minutes

Prep Time: 15 Minutes

Cook Time: 20 Minutes

Ingredients
- 6 ounces tilapia fillets
- 2 teaspoon arrow root
- 1 cup mushrooms, sliced
- 1 clove garlic, finely chopped
- 1 small onion, thinly sliced
- 2 tablespoons extra-virgin olive oil
- ½ cup fresh parsley, roughly chopped
- 1 teaspoon thyme leaves, finely chopped
- ½ cup water
- A pinch of freshly ground black pepper
- A pinch of sea salt

Directions

Preheat your oven to 350°F.

Add extra virgin olive oil to a frying pan set over medium heat; sauté onion, garlic and mushrooms for about 4 minutes or until mushrooms are slightly tender.

Stir in arrowroot, sea salt, thyme and pepper and cook for about 1 minute.

Stir in water until thickened; stir in parsley and cook for 1 minute more.

Place the fillets on a baking tray lined with parchment paper; cover the fish with mushroom sauce and bake for about 20 minutes or until the fish is cooked through.

Nutritional Information per Serving:

Calories: 177; Total Fat: 7.2 g; Carbs: 3.3 g; Dietary Fiber: 1.4 g; Sugars: 1.1 g; Protein: 14.9 g; Cholesterol: 1 mg; Sodium: 66 mg

62. Spiced Roast Side of Salmon

Yield: 6 Servings

Total Time: 30 Minutes

Prep Time: 10 Minutes

Cook Time: 20 Minutes

Ingredients

- 1 tablespoon olive oil
- 1½ kg side of salmon
- 1 teaspoon honey
- 1 tablespoon wholegrain mustard
- ½ teaspoon black peppercorns
- 1 teaspoon paprika
- ½ teaspoon ground ginger
- 1 lemon, cut into wedges

Directions

Preheat your oven to 350 degrees and prepare a roasting tin by lining it with foil. Brush the fish with oil and place in the tin, skin side down.

In a small bowl, mix together a teaspoon of olive oil, honey, mustard, pepper and paprika and then smear the mixture onto the salmon.

Roast the fish in the oven for 20 minutes or until cooked through. Serve with lemon wedges. Enjoy!

Nutritional Information per Serving:

Calories: 482; Total Fat: 30 g; Carbs: 2 g; Dietary Fiber: 0 g; Sugars: 1 g; Protein: 51 g; Cholesterol: 0 mg; Sodium: 400 mg

63. Curried Prawns with White Bread

Yield 4 Servings

Total Time: 1 Hour

Prep Time: 15 Minutes

Cook Time: 25 Minutes

Ingredients
- 225g jumbo prawns, peeled
- 1 cup vegetable stock
- 1 inch ginger root, thinly stripped
- 1 red chili, seeded and thinly sliced
- 1 can coconut milk
- 2 tablespoons hot curry powder
- 75 g sugar snap peas
- 1 large sweet potato, cubed
- Juice of 1 lime
- ½ cup thinly sliced spring onions for serving
- Salt and pepper to taste

Directions

Toast the coconut in a large pan for about 2 minutes until it turn golden. Transfer into a bowl. Return the pan to heat and add curry powder and toast it until fragrant for about a minute then add in the sweet potato cubes, chili and ginger. Pour in the stock and coconut milk and bring to a boil. Lower the heat and simmer for 10 minutes until the potatoes are tender. Stir in the veggies and cook for 5 minutes until soft. Next add the prawns and cook for about 2 minutes or until they turn pink. Season the curry. Turn of the heat and stir in the spring onions and lime juice.

Serve with artisan bread and top with toasted coconut

Nutrition Information per Serving:
Calories: 367,; Total Fat: 16.5 g; Carbs: 33.5 g; Dietary Fiber:1.9 g; Sugar: 13 g; Protein: 26 g; Sodium: 1198 mg; Cholesterol: 112 mg

64. Hot Lemon Garlic Prawns with Rice

Yield: 8 Servings

Total Time: 35 Minutes

Prep Time: 15 Minutes

Cook Time: 20 Minutes

Ingredients
- 1kg raw prawns, peeled, deveined
- 2 cups white rice
- 4 cups water
- ½ teaspoon sea salt
- 2 tablespoons olive oil
- 2 tablespoons coconut oil
- 1 shallot, chopped
- 4 garlic cloves, chopped
- 2 tablespoons minced ginger
- 1/2 teaspoon chilli flakes
- 1/2 teaspoon fennel seeds
- 1 teaspoon ground paprika
- 1/2 cup fresh lemon juice
- 2 tablespoons fresh lemon zest
- 2 tablespoon chopped parsley

Directions

In a large pot, combine olive oil, sea salt and water; stir in white rice and simmer, covered, for about 20 minutes or until rice is cooked through. Remove from heat and fluff with a spoon to cool. Heat coconut oil in a skillet over medium heat and stir in shallots, fennel seeds, and chilli flakes for about 2 minutes or until shallots are tender. Stir in garlic, ginger, paprika and prawns, sea salt and pepper and cook for about 5 minutes or until the prawns are cooked through. Remove the pan from heat and stir in fresh lemon juice, lemon zest and parsley. Serve the prawn and sauce over a bowl of cooked white rice.

Nutritional Information per Servings:
Calories: 311; Total Fat: 12 g; Carbs: 11 g; Dietary Fiber: 2.7 g; Sugars: 3 g; Protein: 15 g; Cholesterol: 189 mg; Sodium: 557 mg

65. White Fish & Coconut Rice

Yield: 4 Servings

Total Time: 40 Minutes

Prep Time: 10 Minutes

Cook Time: 30 Minutes

Ingredients

- 4 (150-gram) skinless Mahi Mahi fillets
- ½ teaspoon paprika
- 1/2 cup fresh lemon juice
- ½ teaspoon sea salt
- ½ teaspoon black pepper
- 4 tablespoons coconut oil
- 4 cups white rice
- 1 cup coconut milk
- Lemon wedges

Directions

Preheat your oven to 385 degrees. Season the Mahi Mahi fish with fresh lemon juice, paprika, sea salt, and black pepper.

Heat a tablespoon of oil in a skillet and sear the seasoned fish for about 3 minutes per side or until golden browned.

Transfer to a baking pan and bake for about 10 minutes or until the fish is cooked through.

Combine coconut milk, salt and olive oil in a pan; stir in rice and cook for about 20 minutes or until rice is cooked through.

Serve the fish with the coconut rice.

66. Grilled Beef & White Rice

Yield: 3 Servings

Total Time: 15 Minutes

Prep Time: 10 Minutes

Cook Time: 5 Minutes

Ingredients
- 350g lean beef steak
- 2 tablespoons freshly squeezed orange juice
- 2 tablespoons freshly squeezed lemon juice
- 2 tablespoons freshly squeezed lime juice
- 3 tablespoons extra-virgin olive oil
- 1 teaspoon raw honey
- 1 teaspoon raw apple-cider vinegar
- ¼ teaspoon coarse salt
- ¼ teaspoon black pepper
- 3 cups cooked white rice

Directions

In a bowl, whisk together the dressing juices, olive oil, honey, apple cider vinegar, salt and pepper until well combined; add in the meat and let marinate for at least 30 minutes.

Preheat your grill on medium heat; grill the steak for about 8 minutes per side or until golden browned on the outside and cooked through.

Let cool and slice into small pieces. Serve with cooked white rice and a glass of juice.

Nutritional Information per Serving:
Calories: 315; Fat: 25.8 g; Carbs: 4.8 g; Dietary Fiber: 1.2 g; Sugars: 1.2 g; Protein: 39.3 g; Cholesterol: 255 mg; Sodium: 581 mg

67. Ginger Chicken with Veggies

Yields: 4 Servings

Total Time: 15 Minutes

Prep Time: 10 Minutes

Cook Time: 5 Minutes

Ingredients

- 2 cup skinless, boneless, and cooked chicken breast meat, diced
- ¼ cup extra virgin olive and canola oil mixture
- 1 teaspoon powdered ginger
- ½ red onion, sliced
- 2 cloves garlic, minced
- ½ bell pepper, sliced
- 1 cup thinly sliced carrots
- ½ cup finely chopped celery
- 1 cup chicken broth (not salted)

Directions

Add the oil mixture to a skillet set over medium heat; sauté onion and garlic until translucent. Stir in the remaining ingredients and simmer for a few minutes or until the veggies are tender.

Nutrition Information per Serving:

Calories: 425; Total Fat: 21.1 g; Carbs: 6.5 g; Dietary Fiber: 1.5 g; Sugars: 3.1 g Protein: 52 g; Cholesterol: 130 mg; Sodium: 301 mg

68. Tasty Coconut Cod

Yields: 4 Servings

Total Time: 35 Minutes

Prep Time: 25 Minutes

Cook Time: 10 Minutes

Ingredients:

- 24 ounces cod fillets, sliced into small strips
- 2 tablespoons coconut oil
- 1 cup finely shredded coconut
- 2 cups coconut milk
- 1 ½ cups coconut flour
- ¼ teaspoon sea salt
- 1 ½ teaspoon ginger powder
- Mango salsa

Directions

Rinse and debone the fish fillets. In a bowl, combine ginger powder, coconut flour and sea salt; set aside. Add coconut milk to another bowl and set aside.

Add shredded coconut to another bowl and set aside. Dip the fillets into coconut milk, then into the flour mixture, back into the milk, and finally into shredded coconut. Add coconut oil to a skillet set over high heat;

when melted and hot, add the fish fillets and cook for about 5 minutes per side or until cooked through.

Serve the cooked cod fillets with mango salsa.

Nutrition Information per Serving:
Calories: 609; Total Fat: 44.3 g; Carbs: 13.2 g; Dietary Fiber: 6.4 g; Sugars: 5.7 g Protein: 43.1 g; Cholesterol: 34 mg; Sodium: 283 mg

69. Lemon BBQ Salmon

Yields: 12 Servings

Total Time: 4 Hours 27 Minutes

Prep Time: 4 Hours 15 Minutes

Cook Time: 12 Minutes

Ingredients

- 12 (180 grams each) Atlantic salmon fillets, with skin on
- 1/2 cup extra virgin olive oil
- 1 bunch roughly chopped lemon thyme
- 1/3 cup finely chopped dill leaves
- 2 tablespoons drained and chopped capers
- 2 fresh lemons, juiced
- 2 garlic cloves, finely chopped
- A pinch of sea salt
- Lemon wedges, to garnish

Directions

In a large jug, mix together lemon thyme, dill, capers, 1/3 cup lemon juice, garlic, extra virgin olive oil, sea salt and pepper. Arrange salmon fillets, in a single layer, in a ceramic dish and pour over half of the marinade. Turn it over and pour over the remaining marinade.

Refrigerate, covered, for about 4 hours. Remove the fish from the refrigerator at least 30 minutes before cooking. Grease barbecue plate and heat on medium high. Barbecue the marinated fish, skin side down, for about 3 minutes. Turn and continue barbecuing, basting occasionally with the marinade, for 6 minutes more or until cooked through. Serve garnished with lemon wedges.

Nutrition Information per Serving:
Calories: 317; Total Fat: 19.6 g; Carbs: 1.9 g; Dietary Fiber: 0.5 g; Sugars: 0.3 g Protein: 35.3 g; Cholesterol: 79 mg; Sodium: 102 mg

CHRON'S DIET SNACKS/DESSERTS

70.   Juice for Gut Health

Yield: 2 Servings

Total Time: 5 Minutes

Prep Time: 5 Minutes

Cook Time: N/A

Ingredients

- 4 stalks of celery
- 1 lemon
- 2 oranges
- 2 apples
- 15 carrots
- Fresh turmeric
- Fresh ginger
- 1 cup coconut water
- pinch of black pepper

Directions

Wash all ingredients and juice through a juicer. Divide between serving glasses and stir in coconut water and black pepper. Enjoy!

71. Raw Banana Mash Snack

Yield: 3 Servings

Total Time: Minutes

Prep Time: 10 Minutes

Cook Time: N/A

Ingredients

- 3 ripe bananas
- 1 cup blueberries
- 1 cup diced apple
- 4 tablespoons almond butter

Directions

Mash bananas in a large bowl; serve topped with the remaining ingredients.

Mash the bananas in a bowl, then top with the remaining ingredients.

Nutrition Information per Serving

Calories: 267; Total Fat: 12.6 g; Carbs: 39.2 g; Dietary Fiber: 7.2 g; Sugars: 23.1 g; Protein: 6 g Cholesterol: 0 mg; Sodium: 3 mg

72. Stomach Soothing Juice

Yield: 1 Serving

Total Time: 10 Minutes

Prep Time: 10 Minutes

Cook Time: N/A

Ingredients

- 3 stalks of celery
- Half of an onion
- 1 clove of garlic
- 1 stalk of broccoli
- 1 grapefruit
- 1 orange
- 1 lemon
- 1 cup elderberries
- 1 teaspoon cinnamon
- 1 teaspoon cayenne pepper
- 1 tablespoon raw honey

Directions

In a blender, blend together all ingredients, except spices and honey. Strain the liquid into a serving glass and stir in cinnamon, cayenne pepper, and raw honey. Enjoy!

73. Sautéed Kale with Citrus Sauce

Yield: 2 Servings

Total Time: 11 Minutes

Prep Time: 5 Minutes

Cook Time: 6 Minutes

Ingredients:

- 1 bunch kale, torn
- 2 tablespoons extra virgin olive oil
- 4 cloves garlic, chopped
- 4 tablespoons fresh orange
- 4 tablespoons fresh lemon juice
- Pinch of sea salt

Directions:

Heat oil in a pan over medium heat; sauté garlic for about 4 minutes or until fragrant. Add kale and cook for about 2 minutes or until wilted; drizzle with fresh orange juice and stir in sea salt. Remove from heat and serve garnished with lemon slices.

Nutrition Information per Serving:
Calories: 163; Total Fat: 14.3 g; Carbs: 8.8 g; Dietary Fiber: 1.3 g; Sugars: 2.8 g Protein: 1.8 g; Cholesterol: 0 mg; Sodium: 139 mg

74. Orange & Aloe Vera Juice

Yield: 2 Servings
Prep Time: 10 Minutes

Ingredients:
- 3 organic oranges
- 2 fresh Aloe Vera branches
- 1 cup mint leaves
- 2-inch fresh ginger root

Directions

Slit the edges of aloe vera with a knife to open the outer layer; scoop out the gel and set aside.
Wash and juice the oranges, mint leaves and ginger. Stir in aloe vera gel and serve right away.

Nutritional info per Serving:
Calories: 164; Total Fat: 0.8 g; Carbs: 39.6 g; Dietary Fiber: 9.9g; Sugars: 27.5 g; Protein: 4.2 g; Cholesterol: 0 mg; Sodium: 52 mg

75. Chocolaty Kamut Energy Bars

Yield: 20 Bars

Total Time: 45 Minutes

Prep Time: 20 Minutes

Cook Time: 25 Minutes

Ingredients:

- 2/3 cup prunes
- 1½ cups water
- ¾ cup coconut
- ¾ cup kamut flour
- 1 cup gluten-free large flake oats
- ½ cup dried cranberries
- ½ cup gluten-free dark chocolate cut into slivers (or chocolate chips)
- ½ cup pumpkin seeds, toasted
- ¼ cup hemp hearts
- 1 banana, mashed
- 3 tbsp. maple syrup

Directions:

Preheat oven to 350°F. Coat a cookie pan with cooking spray and set aside. Combine prunes and water in a pot set over medium high heat; bring to a rolling boil;

remove from heat and let cool for about 10 minutes. Add coconut in a pan set over medium heat; stir for about 3 minutes or until golden brown. Set aside. In a large bowl, combine pumpkin seeds, chocolate, cranberries, oats, flour, and hemp hearts; stir until well combined. Stir in maple syrup and mashed banana.

Transfer the cooked prunes along with cooking water to a food processor and puree until very smooth; add the prune puree to the other ingredients and stir to combine. Transfer the mixture to the pan and bake for about 30 minutes. Remove from oven and let cool before cutting into 20 equal squares. Enjoy!

Nutritional Information per Serving:
Calories: 287; Total Fat: 10.8 g; Carbs: 43.3 g; Dietary Fiber: 5.6 g; Sugars: 18 g; Protein: 6.9 g; Cholesterol: 2 mg; Sodium: 14 mg

76. Gut Friendly Smoothie

Yield: 1 Serving

Total Time: 5 Minutes

Prep Time: 5 Minutes

Cook Time: N/A

Ingredients

- 1 cup of almond milk
- 1/4 cup oats
- 1 banana
- 1 tablespoon cashew nut butter
- 2 thumb fresh ginger
- 1 tablespoon ground turmeric
- 1 teaspoon hemp powder
- 1 teaspoon chia seeds

Directions

Combine all the ingredients in your blender and blend until very smooth. Enjoy!

77. Delicious Mashed Lime Peas

Yield: 2 Servings

Total Time: 10 Minutes

Prep Time: 10 Minutes

Cook Time: N/A

Ingredients

- 2 cups thawed frozen green peas
- ¼ cup fresh lime juice
- 1 teaspoon crushed garlic
- ½ teaspoon cumin
- 1/8 teaspoon hot sauce
- ½ cup chopped cilantro
- 4 green onions, chopped
- 1 tomato, chopped
- Sea salt

Directions

Ina food processor, blend together peas, lime juice, garlic, and cumin until very smooth; transfer to a large bowl and stir in hot sauce, cilantro, green onion, tomato and sea salt. Refrigerate, covered, for about 30 minutes for flavors to blend. Enjoy!

Nutrition Information per Serving
Calories: 137; Total Fat: 0.8 g; Carbs: 25.2 g; Dietary Fiber: 8.8 g; Sugars: 9.9 g; Protein: 8.9 g Cholesterol: 0 mg; Sodium: 90 mg

78. Green Peanut Butter Smoothie

Yield: 1 Serving

Total Time: 5 Minutes

Prep Time: 5 Minutes

Cook Time: N/A

Ingredients

- 1 cup unsweetened almond milk
- ¼ cup oats
- 1 cup fresh spinach
- 1 frozen banana
- ½ teaspoon ground cinnamon
- 1 tablespoon peanut butter

Directions

Combine all the ingredients in your blender and blend until very smooth. Enjoy!

Nutritional Information per Serving:

Calories: 382; Total Fat: 14 g; Carbs: 51 g; Dietary Fiber: 9 g; Sugars: 16 g; Protein: 16 g; Cholesterol: 0 mg; Sodium: 182 mg

79. Delicious Humus

Yield: 6 Servings

Total Time: 10 Minutes

Prep Time: 10 Minutes

Cook Time: N/A

Ingredients

- 2 cloves garlic
- 2 tablespoons sesame seeds, toasted
- 2 tablespoons fresh lemon juice
- 1 cup vegetable broth
- 4 cups cooked garbanzo beans
- ½ cup fresh tarragon leaves, blanched
- 1 cup fresh basil leaves, blanched
- ½ cup fresh parsley
- ¼ cup chopped chives
- Baked potatoes, for serving

Directions

In a food processor, process together all ingredients, except chives and baked potatoes, until very smooth; stir in chives and serve with baked potatoes.

Nutrition Information per Serving

Calories: 523; Total Fat: 10 g; Carbs: 83.5 g; Dietary Fiber: 13.9 g; Sugars: 14.5 g; Protein: 27.9 g Cholesterol: 0 mg; Sodium: 161 mg

80. Easy and Tasty Pumpkin Muffin in a Cup

Yield: 1 Serving

Total Time: 13 Minutes

Prep Time: 10 Minutes

Cook Time: 3 Minutes

Ingredients

- ½ cup homemade pumpkin puree
- 1 tablespoon cacao chocolate chips
- 3/4 cup vegan and gluten free muffin mix
- ½ cup water

Directions

Combine all the ingredients in a microwave-friendly cup until well combined. Pop in the microwave and cook for 3 minutes. Enjoy!

Nutritional Information per Serving:

Calories: 152; Total Fat: 5.4 g; Carbs: 10.3g; Dietary Fiber: 4.1g; Sugars: 6.8 g; Protein: 4.6 g; Cholesterol: 0 mg; Sodium: 4 mg

81. Detoxifying Turmeric Tea

Yield: 1 Serving

Total Time: 10 Minutes

Prep Time: 10 Minutes

Cook Time: N/A

Ingredients

- 1 ½ cups boiling water
- 1 bag of chamomile tea
- 1 bag of peppermint tea
- 1 tablespoon coconut milk
- ½ teaspoon vanilla extract
- 1 teaspoon turmeric
- 1 teaspoon ginger
- 1/4 teaspoon pepper
- 1 teaspoon liquid stevia

Directions

In a large mug, combine hot water, chamomile and peppermint teas and let steep for at least 3 minutes; stir in the remaining ingredients and serve hot!

Nutrition Information per Serving:

Calories: 116; Total Fat: 7 g; Carbs: 13 g; Dietary Fiber: 1 g; Sugars: 2 g Protein: 17 g; Cholesterol: 0 mg; Sodium: 13 mg

82. Green Fruit Drink

Yield: 4 Servings
Total Time: 15 Minutes
Prep Time: 5 Minutes
Cook Time: 10 Minutes

Ingredients

- 3 cups water
- 5 green tea bags
- 1 cup fresh lemon Juice
- 4 drops stevia

Directions

Bring water to a rolling boil; add tea bags and steep for about 4 minutes; strain tea into a pitcher and stir in more water, fresh lemon juice and stevia.

Nutritional Information per Serving:

Calories: 0; Total Fat: 0 g; Carbs: 0 g; Dietary Fiber: 0 g; Sugars: 0 g; Protein: 0 g; Cholesterol: 0 mg; Sodium: 12 mg

83. Superfood Chocolate-Berry Pudding

Yield: 4 Servings

Total Time: 2 Hours

Prep Time: 2 Hours

Cook Time: N/A

Ingredients

- 1/2 cup coconut yogurt
- 2 cups unsweetened coconut milk
- 1/2 cup chia seeds
- 2 tablespoons unsweetened cocoa powder
- 1 teaspoon liquid stevia
- 1/2 cup chopped pistachios
- 1 1/2 cup sliced strawberries
- Mini chocolate chips

Directions

Combine coconut yogurt, coconut mill, chia seeds, cocoa powder and stevia in a blender and blend until smooth; transfer to a bowl and stir in chia seeds. Refrigerate, covered, for at least 2 hours.

When ready to serve, stir well and divide among four serving bowls and layer with sliced strawberries. Top with pistachios and sprinkle with mini chocolate chips and serve.

Nutrition Information per Serving
Calories: 404; Total Fat: 35.6 g; Carbs: 22.9 g; Dietary Fiber: 5.7 g; Sugars: 12.1 g; Protein: 6.1 g Cholesterol: 0 mg; Sodium: 90 mg

84. Fig & Date Coconut Rolls

Yield: 6 Servings

Total Time: 1 Hour

Prep Time: 1 Hour

Cook Time: N/A

Ingredients

- 1 cup walnuts
- 1 cup dried figs
- 1 cup dried dates
- ½ cup fresh shredded coconut

Directions:

Blend together all the ingredients except coconut until the mixture is a smooth paste; roll into small rolls and then roll them into shredded coconut; refrigerate for at least 1 hours before serving.

Nutrition Information per Serving:
Calories: 319; Total Fat: 15 g; Carbs: 46.1 g; Dietary Fiber: 7.6 g; Sugars: 35.3 g; Protein: 7.1 g Cholesterol: 0 mg; Sodium: 6 mg

85. Blissful Matcha-Pistachio Balls

Yield: 4 Servings

Total Time: 20 Minutes

Prep Time: 5 Minutes

Cook Time: N/A

Ingredients

- ½ cup shredded coconut, unsweetened
- 2 Medjool dates, pitted
- ¼ cup raw pistachios, shelled
- ¾ cup raw cashews
- 2 teaspoons matcha powder
- ¼ pistachios, chopped

Directions

In a food processor, process together coconut, dates, cashews, and ¼ cup pistachios, and matcha powder until finely chopped. Roll into small balls and then roll the balls into the remaining chopped pistachios, pressing the pistachios firmly into the balls.

Refrigerate the balls for about 15 minutes before serving.

Nutrition Information per Serving

Calories: 213; Total Fat: 17.9 g; Carbs: 11.4 g; Dietary Fiber: 2.2 g; Sugars: 2.3 g; Protein: 5.4 g Cholesterol: 0 mg; Sodium: 36 mg

86. Savory Coconut Milk & Herb Whole Grain Crackers

Yield: 6 Servings

Total Time: 20 Minutes

Prep Time: 5 Minutes

Cook Time: 15 Minutes

Ingredients:

- 1 cup coconut milk
- 2 teaspoons sesame seeds
- 1 cup whole wheat flour
- 2 teaspoons mixed herbs such as basil and oregano
- ¼ teaspoon sea salt
- ¼ teaspoon pepper

Directions

In a large bowl, whisk together all the ingredients until stiff dough is formed; roll it out into thin chapatis and cut into small strips. Bake them in a 450°F oven for about 15 minutes or until crispy.

Nutrition Information per Serving

Calories: 174; Total Fat: 10.2 g; Carbs: 18.4 g; Dietary Fiber: 1.6 g; Sugars: 1.4 g; Protein: 3.3 g Cholesterol: 0 mg; Sodium: 85 mg

87. Crunchy Veggie Chips

Yield: 8 Serving

Total Time: 19 Minutes

Prep Time: 7 Minutes

Cook Time: 12 Minutes

Ingredients

- 1 cup thinly sliced portobello mushrooms
- 1 cup thinly sliced zucchini
- 1 cup thinly sliced sweet potatoes
- 1 tablespoon extra-virgin olive oil
- Pinch of sea salt
- Pinch of pepper

Directions

Place veggies in a baking dish and drizzle with olive oil; sprinkle with salt and pepper and toss to coat well; bake at 325°F for about 12 minutes or until crunchy. Enjoy!

Nutrition Information per Serving:

Calories: 153; Total Fat: 5 g; Carbs: 24 g; Dietary Fiber: 5 g; Sugars: 7 g Protein: 5 g; Cholesterol: 0 mg; Sodium: 1193 mg

88. Strawberry Sorbet

Yield: 1 Serving

Total Time: 5 Minutes

Prep Time: 5 Minutes

Cook Time: N/A

Ingredients

- 4-6 medium strawberries
- 2 tablespoons fresh lemon juice
- ½ teaspoon vanilla powder
- Flavored stevia
- Ice cubes
- ¼ cup water

Directions

In a blender, blend all ingredients until very smooth; pour into molds and freeze until firm.

Nutritional Information per Serving:
Calories: 26; Total Fat: 0.3 g; Carbs: 4.7 g; Dietary Fiber: 2.7 g; Sugars: 1.7 g; Protein: 1.6 g; Cholesterol: 0 mg; Sodium: 9 mg

89. Dairy-Free Chocolate Mousse

Yield: 3 Servings

Total Time: 10 Minutes

Prep Time: 10 Minutes

Cook Time: N/A

Ingredients:

- 1/2 cup coconut milk
- 1/2 cup cacao powder
- 2 ripe bananas
- 2 ripe avocados
- Pinch of cinnamon
- 1/2 teaspoon vanilla extract
- 1 teaspoon stevia
- Pinch of salt
- Garnish: 1 tablespoon each of toasted hazelnuts, cacao nibs and coconut flakes.

Directions

Combine all ingredients, except garnish, in a food processor and pulse until very smooth. Serve in bowls garnished with toasted hazelnuts, cacao nibs and coconut. Enjoy!

Nutrition Information per Serving:

Calories: 438; Total Fat: 35.9 g; Carbs: 31.9 g; Dietary Fiber: 12 g; Sugars: 11.7 g Protein: 4.3 g; Cholesterol: 0 mg; Sodium: 93 mg

90. Steamed Broccoli and Kalamata Olives

Yield: 2 Servings

Total Time: 15 Minutes

Prep Time: 10 Minutes

Cook Time: 5 Minutes

Ingredients:

- 1 pound broccoli florets
- 1 tablespoon extra-virgin olive oil
- 1 clove garlic, minced
- 12-15 Kalamata olives, sliced in half
- 4 tablespoons fresh lemon juice
- Pinch of sea salt
- Pinch of pepper

Directions

Add broccoli to a steamer basket and bring the water to a rolling boil; steam broccoli for about 5 minutes or until tender crisp. Transfer to a bowl.

Heat oil in a pan and sauté garlic and olives for about 1 minute; stir in broccoli, lemon juice, salt and pepper and serve.

Nutrition Information per Serving:

Calories: 177; Total Fat: 10.8 g; Carbs: 17.9 g; Dietary Fiber: 6.9 g; Sugars: 4.5 g Protein: 6.9 g; Cholesterol: 0 mg; Sodium: 428 mg

91. Sesame Carrots

Yield: 3 Servings

Total Time: 55 Minutes

Prep Time: 10 Minutes

Cook Time: 45 Minutes

Ingredients:

- 1 pound fresh carrots, sliced
- 3 tablespoons sesame oil
- 2 tablespoon sesame seeds
- Pinch of sea salt
- Pinch of pepper

Directions:
Spread carrots in a baking tray and drizzle with 2 tablespoons of sesame oil and toss to coat well; bake, covered, at 400°F for about 30 minutes. Remove from oven and drizzle with remaining sesame oil; sprinkle with salt and pepper and continue baking for about 15 more minutes. Serve sprinkled with toasted sesame seeds. Enjoy!

Nutrition Information per Serving:
Calories: 217; Total Fat: 16.6 g; Carbs: 16.3 g; Dietary Fiber: 4.4 g; Sugars: 7.5 g Protein: 2.3 g; Cholesterol: 0 mg; Sodium: 183 mg

92. Minty-dill Beets

Yield: 3 Servings

Total Time: 40 Minutes

Prep Time: 10 Minutes

Cook Time: 30 Minutes

Ingredients

- 1 pound of beets
- 1 tablespoon extra-virgin olive oil
- sea salt, to taste
- 1 teaspoon dill
- handful of fresh mint

Directions

Boil beets in a pan of salted water for about 40 minutes or until fork tender; remove from heat and let cool. Slice the beets in quarters add to a skillet with olive oil; sprinkle with salt and cook for a few minutes.

Transfer to a bowl and toss in mint and dill. Serve warm.

Nutrition Information per Serving:
Calories: 107; Total Fat: 5 g; Carbs: 15.2; Dietary Fiber: 3.1 g; Sugars: 12 g Protein: 2.6 g; Cholesterol: 0 mg; Sodium: 195 mg

93. Sautéed Kale with Citrus Sauce

Yield: 2 Servings

Total Time: 11 Minutes

Prep Time: 5 Minutes

Cook Time: 6 Minutes

Ingredients:

- 1 bunch kale, torn
- 2 tablespoons extra virgin olive oil
- 4 cloves garlic, chopped
- 4 tablespoons fresh orange
- 4 tablespoons fresh lemon juice
- Pinch of sea salt

Directions:

Heat oil in a pan over medium heat; sauté garlic for about 4 minutes or until fragrant. Add kale and cook for about 2 minutes or until wilted; drizzle with fresh orange juice and stir in sea salt. Remove from heat and serve garnished with lemon slices.

Nutrition Information per Serving:

Calories: 163; Total Fat: 14.3 g; Carbs: 8.8 g; Dietary Fiber: 1.3 g; Sugars: 2.8 g Protein: 1.8 g; Cholesterol: 0 mg; Sodium: 139 mg

94. Spicy Frozen Orange Slices

Yield: 1 Serving

Total Time: 10 Minutes

Prep Time: 10 Minutes

Cook Time: N/A

Ingredients

- 2 tablespoons fresh lemon juice
- Pinch of cardamom
- Pinch of powdered clove
- Pinch of nutmeg
- ¼ teaspoon powdered vanilla
- ¼ teaspoon cinnamon
- Powdered stevia

Directions

Mix stevia with spices; dip oranges into lemon juice and then coat with stevia mix. Freeze until firm.

Nutritional Information per Serving:

Calories: 7; Total Fat: 0.1 g; Carbs: 1.3 g; Dietary Fiber: 0.6 g; Sugars: 0.4 g; Protein: 1.2 g; Cholesterol: 0 mg; Sodium: 10 mg

95. Tasty Fruity Salad

Yield: 4 Servings

Total Time: 5 Minutes

Prep Time: 5 Minutes

Cook Time: N/A

Ingredients

- 1 cup blueberries
- 1 cup diced pineapple
- 1 cup chopped banana
- 1 cup strawberries

Directions

In a large bowl, mix all the ingredients and serve.

Nutritional Information per Serving:
Calories: 86; Total Fat: 0.4 g; Carbs: 22 g; Dietary Fiber: .2 g; Sugars: 14 g; Protein: 1.6 g; Cholesterol: 0 mg; Sodium: 1 mg

96. Healthy Iced Green Tea

Yield: 4 Servings

Total Time: 10 Minutes

Prep Time: 10 Minutes

Cook Time: N/A

Ingredients

- 2 1/2-inch piece fresh ginger, minced
- 3 cups water
- 6 bags green tea
- 3 tablespoons honey
- Mint sprigs, for garnishing

Directions

Combine ginger and 2 water in a saucepan; bring to a gentle boil over medium heat. Lower heat to low and simmer for about 5 minutes. Remove from heat and add the green tea bags and steep for about 3 minutes; strain out the solids and stir in honey.

Add 1 cup of water and chill in the fridge for at least 1 hour. Serve garnished with mint sprigs over ice.

Nutritional Information per Serving:

Calories: 50; Total Fat: 3 g; Carbs: 13 g; Dietary Fiber: 0 g; Protein: 9 g; Cholesterol: 0 mg; Sodium: 10 mg; Sugars: 20.9 g

97. Healthy Green Tea Latte

Yield: 1 Serving

Total Time: 5 Minutes

Prep Time: 5 Minutes

Cook Time: N/A

Ingredients

- 1 teaspoon matcha green tea powder
- 1¾ cup almond milk
- ⅛ teaspoon pure vanilla extract
- 20 drops liquid stevia
- ½ cup ice

Directions

Bend together all ingredients until smooth and frothy. Enjoy!

Nutritional Information per Serving:

Calories: 567; Total Fat: 57.2 g; Carbs: 13.8 g; Dietary Fiber: 6.3 g; Sugars: 8.6 g; Protein: 6.5 g; Cholesterol: 0 mg; Sodium: 40 mg

98. Orange Mint Spritzer

Yield: 2 Servings

Total Time: 5 Minutes

Prep Time: 5 Minutes

Cook Time: N/A

Ingredients

- 1 cup fresh orange juice
- 2 tablespoons raw honey
- Sprigs of mint, chopped
- 2 cups sparkling water

Directions

Mix all ingredients and serve over ice. Enjoy!

Nutritional Information per Serving:
Calories: 240; Total Fat: 0.5 g; Carbs: 60.4 g; Dietary Fiber: 0.6 g; Sugars: 55.3 g; Protein: 1.8 g; Cholesterol: 0 mg; Sodium: 8 mg

99. Chunky monkey smoothie with chia

Ingredients

- 2 tablespoons peanut butter
- 1 frozen banana
- ½ cup Greek yogurt
- 1 cup almond milk
- 2 tablespoons chia seeds

Directions

Combine all the ingredients in your blender and blend until very smooth. Enjoy!

100. Green monster smoothie

Ingredients

- 1 cup Greek yogurt
- 1 Granny Smith apple
- 1 frozen banana
- 1 cup kale
- 1 cup spinach
- 1 cup chopped celery

Directions

Combine all the ingredients in your blender and blend until very smooth. Enjoy!

101. Peachy Coconut Smoothie

Ingredients

- 1 cup frozen peaches
- 1 cup coconut milk
- 2 tablespoons raw honey

Directions
Combine all the ingredients in your blender and blend until very smooth. Enjoy!

102. Banana Pistachio Coconut Smoothie

Ingredients

- 1 cup almond milk
- 2 tablespoons coconut flakes
- 2 tablespoons shelled pistachios
- 1 frozen banana
- 1 tablespoon raw honey

Directions
Combine all the ingredients in your blender and blend until very smooth. Enjoy!

103. Carrot Cake Smoothie

Ingredients

- ½ cup frozen pineapple
- 1 frozen banana
- 1 cup almond milk
- 2 carrots shredded
- 1 pinch nutmeg
- ¼ teaspoon cinnamon
- 2 tablespoons raw honey

Directions

Combine all the ingredients in your blender and blend until very smooth. Enjoy!

Conclusion

Congratulations, after reading and understanding this informative eBook aimed at shedding light on Crohn's disease, you are on the road to digestive health success. You are now fully equipped with the information you need to take care of your body and embrace a natural and healthy diet.

Better still, you not only understand how to diagnose your body's early warning signs that all might not be well but, what you need to do to achieve optimum gut health after diagnosis.

Remember to first see your doctor and follow the guidelines in this book. Feel free to share this information with friends and family that may be suffering from Crohn's disease or other gut-related disease.

You are now on the road to great health. Enjoy and all the best!

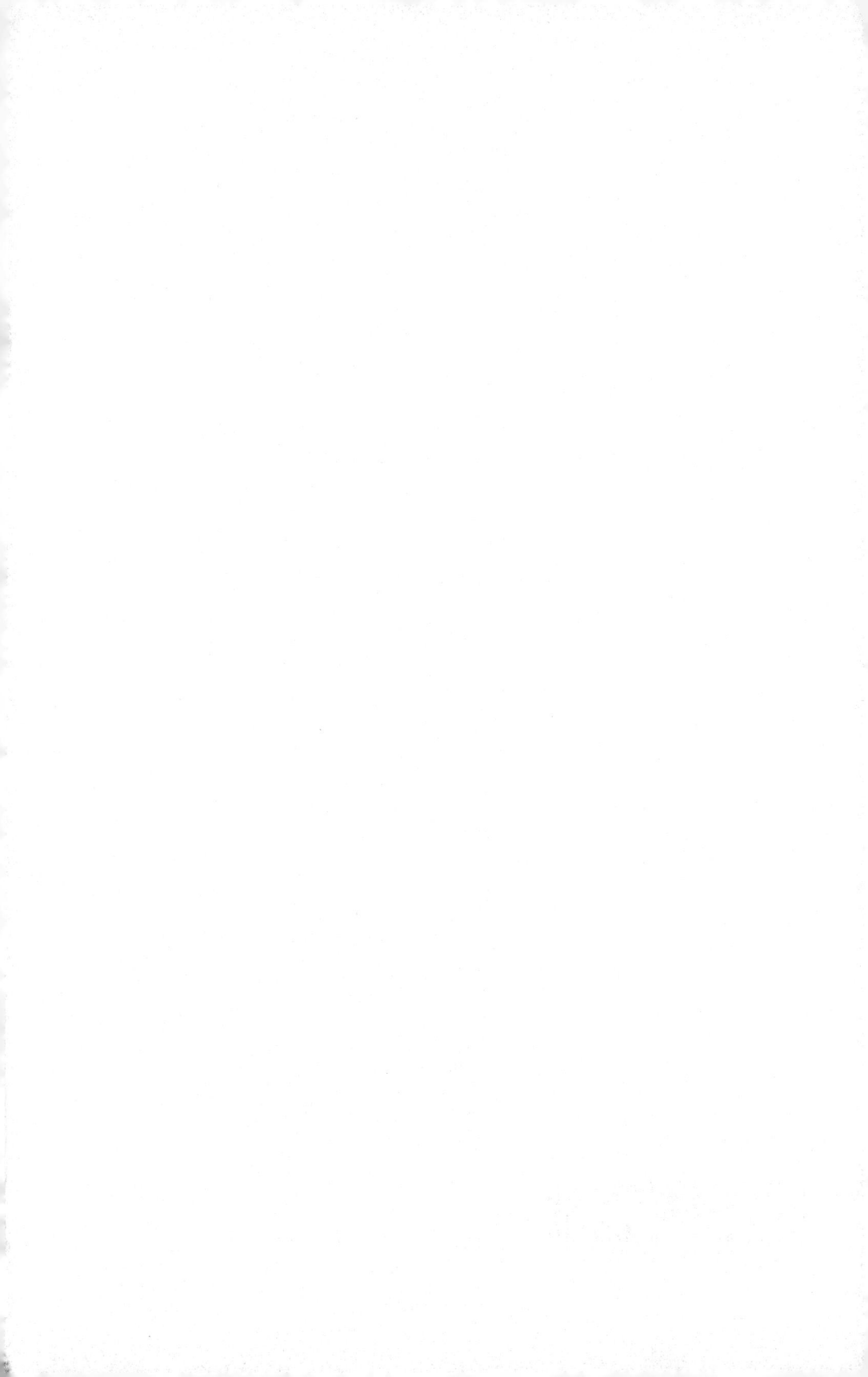

Made in the USA
Middletown, DE
26 April 2021